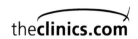

CARDIOLOGY CLINICS

Interventional Cardiology

GUEST EDITOR
Samin K. Sharma, MD

CONSULTING EDITOR
Michael H. Crawford, MD

May 2006 • Volume 24 • Number 2

SAUNDERS

An Imprint of Elsevier, Inc.
PHILADELPHIA   LONDON   TORONTO   MONTREAL   SYDNEY   TOKYO

W.B. SAUNDERS COMPANY
A Division of Elsevier Inc.

Elsevier Inc. • 1600 John F. Kennedy Blvd., Suite 1800 • Philadelphia, Pennsylvania 19103-2899

http://www.theclinics.com

CARDIOLOGY CLINICS	**Volume 24, Number 2**
May 2006	**ISSN 0733-8651**
Editor: Karen Sorensen	**ISBN 1-4160-3521-4**

Reprints. For copies of 100 or more, of articles in this publication, please contact the Commercial Reprints Department, Elsevier Inc., 360 Park Avenue South, New York, New York 10010-1710. Tel. (212) 633-3813 Fax: (212) 462-1935 email: reprints@elsevier.com

The ideas and opinions expressed in *Cardiology Clinics* do not necessarily reflect those of the Publisher. The Publisher does not assume any responsibility for any injury and/or damage to persons or property arising out of or related to any use of the material contained in this periodical. The reader is advised to check the appropriate medical literature and the product information currently provided by the manufacturer of each drug to be administered to verify the dosage, the method and duration of administration, or contraindications. It is the responsibility of the treating physician or other health care professional, relying on independent experience and knowledge of the patient, to determine drug dosages and the best treatment for the patient. Mention of any product in this issue should not be construed as endorsement by the contributors, editors, or the Publisher of the product or manufacturers' claims.

Cardiology Clinics (ISSN 0733-8651) is published quarterly by W.B. Saunders, 360 Park Avenue South, New York, NY 10010-1710. Months of publication are February, May, August, and November. Business and editorial Offices: 1600 John F. Kennedy Blvd., Suite 1800, Philadelphia, PA 19103-2899. Accounting and circulation offices: 6277 Sea Harbor Drive, Orlando, FL 32887-4800. Periodicals postage paid at New York, NY, and additional mailing offices. Subscription prices are $170.00 per year for US individuals, $266.00 per year for US institutions, $85.00 per year for US students and residents, $210.00 per year for Canadian individuals, $323.00 per year for Canadian institutions, $230.00 per year for international individuals, $323.00 per year for international institutions and $115.00 per year for Canadian and foreign students/residents. To receive student/resident rate, orders must be accompanied by name of affiliated institution, data of term, and the *signature* of program/residency coordinator on institution letterhead. Orders will be billed at individual rate until proof of status is received. Foreign air speed delivery is included in all *Clinics* subscription prices. All prices are subject to change without notice. POSTMASTER: Send address changes to *Cardiology Clinics*, Elsevier Periodicals Customer Service, 6277 Sea Harbor Drive, Orlando, FL 32887-4800. **Customer Service: 1-800-654-2452 (US). From outside of the US, call 1-407-345-1000.**

Cardiology Clinics is also published in Spanish by McGraw-Hill Interamericana Editores S. A., P.O. Box 5-237, 06500, Mexico D. F., Mexico; in Portuguese by Reichmann and Alfonso Editores Rio de Janeiro, Brazil; and in Greek by Dimitrios P. Lagos, 8 Pondon Street, GR115-28 Ilissia, Greece.

Cardiology Clinics is covered in *Index Medicus, Excerpta Medica, The Cumulative Index to Nursing and Allied Health Literature* (INAHL).

Printed in the United States of America.

CONSULTING EDITOR

MICHAEL H. CRAWFORD, MD, Professor of Medicine, Lucie Stern Chair in Cardiology, University of California, San Francisco; Chief of Clinical Cardiology, University of California, San Francisco Medical Center, San Francisco, California

GUEST EDITOR

SAMIN K. SHARMA, MD, FACC, Director, Cardiac Catheterization Laboratory & Interventional Cardiology, New York; Zena and Michael A. Wiener Professor of Medicine, New York; and Co-director, Cardiovascular Institute, Mount Sinai Hospital, New York, New York

CONTRIBUTORS

NITIN BARMAN, MD, Interventional Cardiology Fellow, Department of Cardiovascular Medicine, Mount Sinai Hospital, New York, New York

DEEPAK L. BHATT, MD, Staff, Cardiac, Peripheral, and Carotid Intervention, Associate Professor of Medicine, Department of Cardiovascular Medicine, The Cleveland Clinic Foundation, Cleveland, Ohio

GREGORY A. BRADEN, MD, Director of Cardiac Catheterization Laboratory; Director of Cardiovascular Research, Syth Medical Center; Cardiology Specialists of North Carolina, Winston-Salem, North Carolina

VICTOR CHEN, MBChB, FRACP, Interventional Cardiology Fellow, Cardiac Catheterization Laboratory, Cardiovascular Institute, Mount Sinai Hospital, New York, New York

JOAQUIN E. CIGARROA, MD, Department of Internal Medicine, Cardiovascular Division, University of Texas Southwestern Medical Center, Dallas, Texas

L. DAVID HILLIS, MD, Department of Internal Medicine, Cardiovascular Division, University of Texas Southwestern Medical Center, Dallas, Texas

MICHAEL C. KIM, MD, FACC, Director, Coronary Care Unit; Assistant Professor of Medicine, The Cardiovascular Institute, The Mount Sinai School of Medicine, New York, New York

ANNAPOORNA S. KINI, MD, MRCP, FACC, Associate Professor, Department of Medicine; Associate Director, Cardiac Catheterization Laboratory; Director, Interventional Cardiology Fellowship Program, Mount Sinai Hospital, New York, New York

WARREN K. LASKEY, MD, Division Chief, Department of Medicine, Division of Cardiology, University of New Mexico School of Medicine, Albuquerque, New Mexico

MICHAEL S. LEE, MD, Interventional Cardiologist, Cardiovascular Intervention Center, Cedars-Sinai Medical Center, University of California, Los Angeles School of Medicine, Los Angeles, California

RAJ R. MAKKAR, MD, Interventional Cardiologist, Cardiovascular Intervention Center, Cedars-Sinai Medical Center, University of California, Los Angeles School of Medicine, Los Angeles, California

STEPHEN J. NICHOLLS, MBBS, PhD, Research Fellow, Interventional Cardiology, Department of Cardiovascular Medicine, The Cleveland Clinic Foundation, Cleveland, Ohio

JEFFREY J. POPMA, MD, Director, Interventional Cardiology, Associate Professor of Medicine, Department of Internal Medicine (Cardiovascular Division), Brigham and Women's Hospital, Boston, Massachusetts

SAMIN K. SHARMA, MD, FACC, Director, Cardiac Catheterization Laboratory & Interventional Cardiology; Zena and Michael A. Wiener Professor of Medicine; and Co-director, Cardiovascular Institute, Mount Sinai Hospital, New York, New York

ILKE SIPAHI, MD, Research Fellow, Intravascular Ultrasound Core Laboratory, Department of Cardiovascular Medicine, The Cleveland Clinic Foundation, Cleveland, Ohio

RICHARD L. SNIDER, MD, Cardiology Fellow, Department of Medicine, Division of Cardiology, University of New Mexico School of Medicine, Albuquerque, New Mexico

MARK TULLI, MD, Interventional Cardiology Fellow, Department of Internal Medicine (Cardiovascular Division), Brigham and Women's Hospital, Boston, Massachusetts

E. MURAT TUZCU, MD, Professor of Medicine, Cleveland Clinic Lerner College of Medicine, Case Western Reserve University, Cleveland, Ohio; and Medical Director, Intravascular Ultrasound Core Laboratory, Department of Cardiovascular Medicine, The Cleveland Clinic Foundation, Cleveland, Ohio

CONTRIBUTORS

CONTENTS

pharmacologic agents and includes a discussion of the more promising potential future therapies. The clinical trials that provide the basis for the current standard of care are provided, as are ongoing trials that will likely shape the future standard. This article is not intended to provide a detailed discussion of precise mechanistic or structural features of each agent but to serve as a practical clinical guide to the interventionalist when choosing specific pharmacotherapies for specific patients in the catheterization laboratory.

With increased operator experience and improved device technology, there has been a constant growth in the number of complex lesions (ie, thrombotic lesions, diffuse lesions, calcified lesions, nondilatable rigid lesions, ostial lesions, bifurcations, and chronic total occlusions) attempted by interventionalists with the use of drug-eluting stents. Although coronary stent implantation remains the mainstay and ultimate step for the treatment of most coronary lesions, adjunctive devices may be essential for lesion preparation in some cases (5%-10%) to allow stent deployment and expansion and prevent distal embolization. Thrombectomy and distal protection devices have shown to be effective in the interventions of saphenous vein graft lesions, although their use remains unproven in acute myocardial infarctions.

Percutaneous coronary intervention has evolved dramatically over the past 25 years as coronary stents replaced stand-alone balloon angioplasty. Improvements in stents were made in the 1990s, but a breakthrough occurred in early 2000 with the development of stents that eluted pharmacology agents directly into the vessel wall by means of a controlled release from a durable polymer coating. Various drug-eluting stents were developed, each varying with its delivery platform, polymer coating (or absence of coating), and drug selected for elution. This article describes the clinically available and late developmental drug-eluting stent programs targeted for treating patients who have coronary artery disease.

Treatment of coronary bifurcation lesions represents a challenging area in interventional cardiology, but recent advances in percutaneous coronary interventions have led to a dramatic increase in the number of patients successfully treated percutaneously. When compared with nonbifurcation interventions, bifurcation interventions have a lower rate of procedural success, higher procedural costs, longer hospitalization, and a higher rate of clinical and angiographic restenosis. The recent introduction of drug-eluting stents has resulted in a lower event rate and reduction of main vessel restenosis compared with historical controls. Side branch ostial residual stenosis and long-term restenosis remain a problem, however. Although stenting the main vessel with provisional side branch stenting seems to be the prevailing approach, in the era of drug-eluting stents, various two-stent techniques have emerged to allow stenting of the large side branch also.

Chronic total coronary occlusions (CTO) occur in up to one-third of patients undergoing coronary angiography. Indications for opening CTOs include relief of angina, improving left ventricular function, decreasing the need for coronary artery bypass surgery, and improved long-term survival. Newer technology, wire-based and non–wired-based, has improved the ability to cross these previously uncrossable lesions, thereby improving the acute success rates of opening these lesions. Also, the advent of drug-eluting stents has markedly increased the long-term patency of these complex lesions. Therefore, the clinical demand for opening these chronically occluded arteries has increased.

FORTHCOMING ISSUES

RECENT ISSUES

ELSEVIER
SAUNDERS

CARDIOLOGY
CLINICS

Cardiol Clin 24 (2006) ix

Foreword

Interventional Cardiology

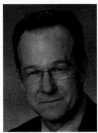

Michael H. Crawford, MD
Consulting Editor

Interventional cardiology has moved from coronary angioplasty to percutaneous interventions on the heart and vasculature. This issue of *Cardiology Clinics* focuses on coronary artery interventions. We are fortunate to have Dr. Samin Sharma, who directs one of the premier cardiac interventional laboratories in the United States, as guest editor for this issue. He and his colleagues have contributed a great deal to the advancement of the technical aspects of coronary interventions. They and other experts from the United States have put together an outstanding comprehensive discussion of current issues in coronary interventions, including a discussion of who should have a percutaneous coronary intervention and safety concerns.

The appropriate application of any technology is often its Achilles' heel. Being accomplished at doing something does not necessarily translate to having good judgment about when to use this skill. Ideally good judgment is developed over time; hence the development of interventional cardiology training programs, boards, and the special certificate in this subdiscipline of cardiology. With coronary artery bypass surgery providing

very similar outcomes, patient selection in more challenging patients is crucial. Also, advances in the management of cardiovascular disease and heightened expectations of patients are bringing many 80- and 90-year-olds who have advanced vascular disease to the catheterization laboratory. Although bypass surgery seems overly aggressive and is often not welcomed in such patients, one must be able to comprehend the limits of percutaneous interventions also. Many difficult situations confront the interventional cardiologist today, and this issue of *Cardiology Clinics* provides an excellent database for approaching management decisions in patients who have coronary artery disease.

Michael H. Crawford, MD
Division of Cardiology
Department of Medicine
University of California, San Francisco Medical
Center
505 Parnassus Avenue, Box 0124
San Francisco, CA 94143, USA

E-mail address: crawafordm@medicine.ucsf.edu

Preface

Interventional Cardiology

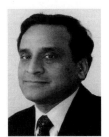

Samin K. Sharma, MD
Guest Editor

Since the introduction of balloon angioplasty by Andreas Gruentzig in 1977, interventional cardiology has immensely proliferated in the last three decades. In 2005, approximately 1.2 million percutaneous coronary interventional (PCI) procedures were performed in the United States, and about 2 million were performed worldwide. This unprecedented exponential growth in interventional cardiology has been possible because of (1) continued refinement in technique and the advent of new devices to improve the success and safety of PCI, (2) expanded indications by well-defined randomized clinical trials, and (3) dramatically reduced rates of restenosis by the advent of drug-eluting stents (DES). Despite the increasing complexity of cases, the outcome of PCI has continued to improve, and selected cases are being done on an ambulatory basis. The need for urgent bypass surgery resulting from PCI complications has been almost eliminated, pushing this field further by allowing freestanding catherization laboratories to perform PCI without on-site surgery. Interventional cardiologists have now expanded their skills outside the realm of coronary tree to include noncoronary vascular interventions: carotids, subclavian, renal, iliac, among others.

This issue of *Cardiology Clinics* has compiled a group of world-class authors to provide the most updated view in this ever-changing and growing field of interventional cardiology. Important topics such as lesion classification, intravascular ultrasound, current antiplatelet therapy, and vascular closure devices are presented in a practical manner. Lesion-specific approaches using various debulking and thrombectomy devices, bifurcation lesions, and total occlusions are discussed in detail with practical tips. The section on DES provides the update of various DES program and trial results. The controversies of PCI versus coronary artery bypass grafting along with recent PCI guidelines are outlined in a fairly balanced overview. Finally, quality issues in the catheterization laboratory have been emphasized to continue to do the best safely.

I am indebted to all the authors who have made possible this world-class handbook for the interventional cardiologists, fellows, and support staff. Undoubtedly it will serve as an important reference resource for those who are participating in the field of interventional cardiology. I wish to thank my colleagues and staff of the Cardiac Catheterization Laboratory who have helped refine the overall care of cardiac interventional patients at the Mount Sinai Hospital, making it one of the premier institutions in the state.

Samin K. Sharma, MD
Cardiac Catheterization Laboratory &
Interventional Cardiology
Mount Sinai Hospital
One Gustave L. Levy Place, Box 1030
New York, NY 10029, USA

E-mail address: samin.sharma@msnyuhealth.org

0733-8651/06/$ - see front matter © 2006 Elsevier Inc. All rights reserved.
doi:10.1016/j.ccl.2006.04.010

Coronary Angiography, Lesion Classification and Severity Assessment

Annapoorna S. Kini, MD, MRCP

*Cardiac Catheterization Laboratory, Cardiovascular Institute, Mount Sinai Hospital,
Box 1030, One Gustave Place, New York, NY 10029, USA*

Advances in the technique of coronary intervention over the years have changed the management of patients with coronary artery disease, resulting in safer and more effective percutaneous revascularization in patients previously deemed at high risk for nonsurgical approaches. Angiographic factors contributing to an untoward procedural outcome after coronary revascularization have been characterized, and a lesion complexity score has been developed. Recognition of these angiographic risk factors has proven invaluable for triaging patients to coronary intervention, coronary bypass surgery, or medical therapy. The post-treatment lumen diameter has been the most important predictor of late clinical and angiographic recurrence after coronary revascularization in several single and multi-center clinical trials. Coronary angiography (visual or quantitative) is a simple, easy, and mostly reliable tool for assessing lesion severity, but it may be inconclusive in the borderline lesions (40% to 60% diameter obstruction). Anatomical (using intravascular ultrasound) and physiological (using coronary flow reserve or fractional flow reserve) lesion assessment may be required for adequate lesion evaluation, before and after percutaneous coronary intervention (PCI).

Lesion classification

Coronary lesion classification is based most commonly on American College of Cardiology/American Heart Association (ACC/AHA) task

force classification, along with other recent classifications [1].

The American College of Cardiology/American Heart Association task force on lesion morphology

A joint task force of the ACC and the AHA established criteria in 1988 to estimate procedural success and complication rates after balloon angioplasty, based on the presence or absence of specific lesion characteristics (Box 1) [2]. Although these criteria were developed based solely upon the task force's clinical impressions in the era of balloon angioplasty, the estimates of procedural success and complications were correlated closely with the procedural outcomes subsequently demonstrated in patients undergoing multi-vessel coronary angioplasty or stenting. Procedural success and complication rates were 92% and 2%, respectively, for type A lesions; 76% and 10%, respectively, for type B lesions; and 61% and 21%, respectively, for type C lesions. Lesions with two or more type B characteristics (modified ACC/AHA type B2) had an intermediate risk between lesions with one type B characteristic (modified ACC/AHA type B1) and type C lesions. Most of the studies have categorized B2 and C lesion types as complex or high-risk lesion characteristics. Specific lesion characteristics associated with an adverse outcome included chronic total occlusion, high-grade stenosis, stenosis on a bend of 60 degrees or more, and lesions located in vessels with proximal tortuosity.

Despite the advantages of this composite approach for estimating lesion complexity, the ACC/AHA classification system has certain limitations. The definitions used in the classification

E-mail address: annapoorna.kini@msnyuhealth.org

0733-8651/06/$ - see front matter © 2006 Elsevier Inc. All rights reserved.
doi:10.1016/j.ccl.2006.04.002

Box 1. Characteristics of type A, B and C coronary lesions as per American College of Cardiology/American Heart Association classification

Type A lesion (high success, greater than 85%; low risk)
- Discrete (less than 10 mm)
- Little or no calcium
- Concentric
- Less than totally occlusive
- Readily accessible
- Not ostial in location
- Nonangulated segment, less than 45°
- No major side branch involvement
- Smooth contour
- Absence of thrombus

Type B lesions (moderate success, 60% to 85%; moderate risk)
- Tubular (10 to 20 mm length)
- Moderate to heavy calcification
- Eccentric
- Total occlusions less than 3 months old
- Moderate tortuosity of proximal segment
- Ostial in location
- Moderately angulated segment, at least 45°, less than 90°
- Bifurcation lesion requiring double guidewire
- Irregular contour
- Some thrombus present

Type C lesions (low success, less than 60%; high risk)
- Diffuse (at least 2 cm length)
- Total occlusion more than 3 months old
- Excessive tortuosity of proximal segment
- Inability to protect major side branches
- Extremely angulated segments at least 90°
- Degenerated vein grafts with friable lesions

system (eg, lesion eccentricity, irregularity, angulation, and tortuosity) are subject to individual interpretations. As a result, considerable observer variability has been reported. Some ACC/AHA lesion features are associated with a complicated procedure (eg, thrombus and angulated segments), whereas others are associated with an unsuccessful but uncomplicated procedure (eg, old total occlusions or longer lesions). Owing to the heterogeneity of the morphologic features within this classification system, its generalized use in estimating procedural outcome for all patients may be problematic. Various preprocedural lesion morphologies have been outlined in Box 2.

Angulated lesions

Vessel curvature at the site of maximum stenosis should be measured in the most unforeshortened projection using a length of curvature that approximates the balloon length used for coronary dilation. Percutaneous interventions of highly angulated (at least 45°) lesions have been associated with an increased risk of procedural complications (13% versus 3.5% in nonangulated stenoses, $P < .001$), most commonly owing to coronary dissection.

Bifurcation lesions

The risk of side branch (SB) occlusion in bifurcation lesions relates to the extent of atherosclerotic involvement of the SB within its origin from the parent vessel (14% to 27% in SB with ostial involvement). To accurately assess the risk of SB occlusion and avoid conflicting definitions of SB and ostial stenoses, few classifications were accepted, most used being Duke classification (Fig. 1).

Lesion calcification

Angiographic and intravascular studies have shown that the presence of coronary artery calcium is an important marker for coronary atherosclerosis. The presence of coronary artery calcium also has been related to reduced procedural success rates after coronary interventions, in part because of lesion rigidity, development of dissections at calcified plaque-normal wall interface, and the inability of the atherectomy cutting chamber to excise the fibrocalcific plaque. In contrast, higher (greater than 90%) procedural success rates have been reported after rotational atherectomy (an atheroablative device creates microdissection planes within the fibrocalcific plaque and allows more effective arterial expansion after balloon angioplasty or stent placement).

Despite the prognostic importance of lesion calcium on procedural outcome after coronary intervention, conventional angiography has been

---

Box 2. Definitions of preprocedural lesion morphology

Lesion angulation—vessel angle formed by the center line through the lumen proximal to the stenosis and extending beyond it and a second center line in the straight portion of the artery distal to the stenosis
- Moderate—lesion angulation at least 45°
- Severe—lesion angulation at least 90°

Calcification—readily apparent densities noted within the apparent vascular wall at the site of the stenosis
- Moderate—densities noted only with cardiac motion prior to contrast injection
- Severe—radiopacities noted without cardiac motion prior to contrast injection

Eccentricity—stenosis that is noted to have one of its luminal edges in the outer one quarter of the apparently normal lumen

Filling defect—an angiographic lucency, usually globular, with contrast surrounding at least 3 sides (or equivalent), divided into three grades: 1 = haziness alone, 2 = defect 1 to 2 mm, 3 = defect greater than 2 mm in diameter

Irregularity—characterized by lumen ulceration, intimal flap, aneurysm, or sawtooth pattern
- Ulceration—lesions with a small crater consisting of a discrete luminal widening in the area of the stenosis is noted, provided it does not extend beyond the normal arterial lumen
- Intimal flap—a mobile, radiolucent extension of the vessel wall into the arterial lumen
- Aneurismal dilation—segment of arterial dilation larger than the dimensions of the normal arterial segment
- Sawtooth pattern—multiple, sequential stenosis irregularities

Lesion angle—degrees at end diastole in nonforeshortened view subtended by a 15 mm treatment device

Lesion ectasia—at least 150% of reference diameter

Lesion length—measured shoulder-to-shoulder in an unforeshortened view
- Discrete—lesion length less than 10 mm
- Tubular—lesion length 10 to 20 mm
- Diffuse—lesion length at least 20 mm

Ostial location—origin of the lesion within 3 mm of the vessel origin

Total occlusion—TIMI 0 or 1 flow

Nonchronic total occlusion—total occlusion not meeting the criteria for chronicity

Thrombus—discrete, intraluminal filling defect is noted with defined borders and is separated largely from the adjacent wall. Contrast staining may or may not be present.

Bifurcation stenosis—present if a medium or large branch (greater than 1.5 mm) originates within the stenosis and if the side branch is surrounded completely by stenotic portions of the lesion to be dilated

Lesion accessibility (proximal tortuosity)
- Moderate tortuosity—lesion is distal to two bends at least 75°
- Severe tortuosity—lesion is distal to three bends at least 75°

Degenerated saphenous vein graft—graft characterized by luminal irregularities or ectasia comprising more than 50% of the graft length

---

shown to have limited sensitivity for detecting smaller amounts of calcium within the coronary artery.

Degenerated saphenous vein grafts

Few criteria have been proposed for classifying the degree of graft degeneration, although such a definition should include an estimate of the percentage of graft irregularity and ectasia, friability, presence of thrombus, and number of discrete or diffuse lesions (greater than 50% stenosis) located within the graft. These pathologic features have been correlated clinically with graft atherosclerosis and may predispose to distal microembolization, thrombosis, and other

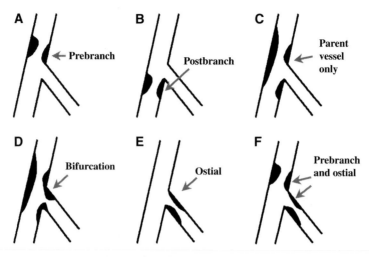

Fig. 1. Bifurcation lesion classification.

complications during saphenous vein graft intervention.

Eccentric lesions

Pathologic studies have demonstrated that balloon angioplasty of eccentric lesions may result in the asymmetric expansion of normal vessel wall, with little change to the underlying atherosclerotic segment. Historically, reduced procedural success rates have been attributed to eccentric lesions, presumably owing to greater degrees of elastic recoil and larger residual percent diameter stenoses in these lesions.

Inaccessible lesions

The vessel tortuosity is assessed before the lesion that is going to be treated percutaneously (Fig. 2).

Irregular lesions

Lesion irregularity includes those narrowings with ulceration, aneurysms proximal or distal to stenoses, sawtoothed contour suggesting a friable lesion, and intimal flaps. The presence of lesion irregularity correlates pathologically with plaque fissuring, rupture, and platelet and fibrin aggregation. Accordingly, complex, irregular plaques have been associated with unstable coronary syndromes and progression to total occlusion, whereas smooth lumen contours are more suggestive of stable angina. Other surface morphology features associated with unstable angina and infarction include lesion ulceration, sharply angulated leading or trailing borders, multiple serpiginous channels, and discrete intraluminal filling defects. A qualitative scoring index for lesion irregularity was proposed in 1985, classifying lesions as:

- Concentric (symmetric narrowing)
- Type I eccentric (asymmetric narrowing with a broad neck)
- Type II eccentric (asymmetric narrowing with a narrow neck related to one or more overhanging edges or scalloped borders)
- Multiple irregular coronary narrowings in series

Type II eccentric narrowings were more common in patients with unstable angina, whereas concentric and type I eccentric narrowings were demonstrated more often in those with stable angina.

Long lesions

Several criteria have been used to assess the axial length of the atherosclerotic obstruction in patients undergoing percutaneous coronary intervention. Lesion length may be estimated as the shoulder-to-shoulder extent of atherosclerotic narrowing greater than 20% or by the lesion length with greater than 50% visual diameter stenosis. Sequential stenoses may be included in the estimation of lesion length, provided that the

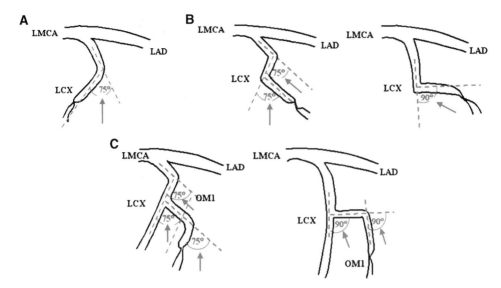

Fig. 2. Assessment of lesion tortuosity. (*A*) No tortuosity or mild tortuosity: no bend or one 75° bend before lesion. (*B*) Moderate tortuosity: two bends of 75° before the lesion or one 90° bend before the lesion. (*C*) Excessive tortuosity: more than two bends of 75° before the lesion or more than one 90° bend before the lesion.

distance between the sequential lesions does not exceed 5 mm.

Ostial lesions

Balloon angioplasty of aorto–ostial lesions and lesions involving the proximal 3 mm of left anterior descending coronary artery (LAD) or left circumflex coronary artery (LCX) has been associated with an unfavorable procedural outcome, potentially owing to smooth muscle and eccentric intimal proliferation noted pathologically in ostial lesions. Technical factors accounting for the suboptimal success rates included difficulties with guide catheter support, lesion inelasticity precluding maximal balloon inflation, and the need for multiple balloon exchanges. Clinical restenosis developed in nearly 50% of patients over the subsequent 6 months. Although directional, rotational, and extractional atherectomy; intracoronary stenting; and excimer laser coronary angioplasty have been used in patients with ostial lesions, late clinic recurrence still may be problematic in this location.

Total occlusion

Total coronary occlusion generally is identified on the cineangiogram as an abrupt termination of the epicardial vessel; anterograde and retrograde collaterals may be present and are helpful in quantifying the length of the totally occluded segment. The risk of an unsuccessful procedure relates to the duration of the occlusion and certain lesion morphologic features, such as bridging collaterals, occlusion length greater than 15 mm, occlusion duration greater than 3 months, and the absence of a nipple to guide wire advancement.

Thrombus

The presence of angiographic thrombus, generally identified by the appearance of discrete, intraluminal filling defects within the arterial lumen, also has been associated with a higher, although widely variable (6% to 73%), incidence of ischemic complications after coronary intervention, primarily resulting from the occurrence of distal embolization and thrombotic occlusions. Although antithrombotic and thrombolytic agents and mechanical devices have been recommended for selected thrombus-containing lesions, it often has been difficult to quantitate the incremental benefit achieved with these techniques over conventional methods.

Thrombus grades

There are six thrombus grades:

- Grade 0—no thrombus
- Grade 1—possible thrombus = mural opacities

- Grade 2—mall thrombus = size < 0.5 × normal lumen diameter
- Grade 3—medium thrombus = size 0.5–1.5 × normal lumen diameter
- Grade 4—large thrombus = size > 1.5 × normal lumen diameter
- Grade 5—recent thrombotic occlusion = fresh thrombus with dye stasis and delayed washout
- Grade 6—chronic total occlusion = smooth, abrupt, and with no dye stasis and brisk flow

Other lesion classifications

Society for Cardiac Angiography and Interventions
The Society for Cardiac Angiography and Interventions (SCAI) [3] lesion classification system divided ACC/AHA lesions into type I to IV:

- Type I lesions (highest success, lowest risk)—patent and do not meet criteria for C lesions
- Type II lesions—patent and meet any of the criteria for ACC/AHA type C lesions
- Type III lesions—occluded and do not meet criteria for C lesions
- Type IV lesions—occluded and meet any of the criteria for ACC/AHA type C lesions (Box 3).

Ellis classification
With newer device strategy and use of dual antiplatelet therapy and intravenous GP IIb/IIIa inhibitors [4], major complications of coronary interventions have declined significantly. Hence a newer scheme to update lesion classification based on the lesion outcome of over 10,000 patients was suggested by Ellis and colleagues [5]. Nonchronic total occlusion (total occlusion not meeting criteria for chronicity) had the highest odds ratio [4.75 (2.69 to 8.38, $P < .001$)] on multivariate analysis to predict periprocedural complications, along with degenerated vein graft lesions.

The strongest correlation was with nonchronic total occlusion with degenerated saphenous vein graph. There was a moderately strong correlation with:

- Lesion length of at least 10 mm
- Lumen irregularities or saw tooth
- Lumen edges in absence of thrombus
- Filling defect greater than 2 mm in diameter
- Calcification

Box 3. American College of Cardiology/ Society for Cardiac Angiography and Interventions lesion classification system

Type I lesions (highest success expected, lowest risk)
Does not meet criteria for ACC/AHA type C lesion
Nontotal occlusion

Type II lesions
Meets any of these criteria for ACC/AHA type C lesion:
- Diffuse (greater than 20 mm length)
- Excessive tortuosity of proximal segment
- Extremely angulated segments, greater than 90°
- Inability to protect major SB
- Degenerated vein grafts with friable lesions
Nontotal occlusion

Type III lesions
Does not meet criteria for type C lesion
Total occlusion

Type IV lesions
Meets any of these criteria for ACC/AHA C lesion:
- Diffuse (greater than 2 cm length)
- Excessive tortuosity of proximal segment
- Extremely angulated segments, greater than 90°
- Inability to protect major SB
- Degenerated vein grafts with friable lesions
- Occluded for more than 3 months
Total occlusion

- Lesion angle of at least 45°
- Eccentricity
- SVG age of at least 10 years

Based on these correlates and PCI outcomes, lesions were divided further as:

- Class I (low risk)—no risk factors
- Class II (moderate)—one to two moderate correlates and absence of strong correlations
- Class III (high risk)—at least three moderate correlates and absence of strong correlates

• Class IV (highest risk)—either of strongest correlates.

Evaluation of lesion severity

Quantitative coronary angiography

Generally, there is good agreement among interventional cardiologists who visually estimate stenosis severity regarding the severity of mild or severe stenosis. In contrast, there is a great deal of intraobserver and interobserver variability regarding intermediate stenosis. In addition, there is some variability in the visual estimate of vessel dimensions. Computer-assisted methods have been developed to provide a more accurate and unbiased assessment of absolute and relative coronary artery dimensions during angiography, a technique called quantitative coronary angiography (QCA). QCA entails digitization of the film, image calibration, arterial contour editing, and observer editing. In addition to the inherent shortcomings of individual QCA systems, there are errors common to all systems at each stage (ie, image acquisition and analysis may be performed during systole, thus skewing the results). Moreover, observer editing may render this objective technique operator-dependent and susceptible to bias. The major advantage of coronary angiography over other techniques of lesion assessment is the ability to assess the severity of the lesion without the need to cross the lesion with a guidewire or other devices.

Pitfalls of coronary angiography

The angiographic assessment of coronary artery lesions is based on the comparison of radiocontrast dye opacification of the lesion relative to a presumed normal reference segment. The true lumen diameter of the reference segment, however, may be measured inaccurately, because it is diseased diffusely and concentrically. Likewise, if the true dimensions of the vessel are underestimated, undersized balloon and stents may be selected for coronary intervention, resulting in suboptimal results and use of additional equipment [6].

Also, because of vascular remodeling, the vessel dimensions at the site of stenosis may change over time relative to the reference segment. The vessel may shrink or grow in diameter focally at the site of stenosis.

Another pitfall of coronary angiography may stem from the eccentricity of the lesion. Even using multiple planar views, it is often difficult to fully delineate the lesion, especially in the presence of ostial or bifurcation lesions or overlapping branches. Therefore, the lesion may be much more severe than appreciated angiographically.

Coronary angiography also may fail to characterize the composition of the atheroma accurately, which is an important factor in the choice of the device used in a possible intervention. For example, calcifications and intracoronary thrombi often produce the same angiographic picture. A heavily calcified lesion may be more suitable for rotational atherectomy, whereas a lesion with a large thrombus burden would contraindicate rotational atherectomy and would be dealt with better with thrombectomy devices.

Intravascular ultrasound

Intravascular ultrasound (IVUS) has become the gold standard for delineating vessel wall anatomy and plaque morphology [7]. Current IVUS catheters with an outer diameter of between 2 to 3 Fr can be introduced by means of 6 Fr guiding catheters. The catheter is placed distal to the segment of interest and is pulled back gradually. Motorized pull-back devices are available, enabling three-dimensional reconstruction of the vessel wall. In many large prospective series, in approximately 20% of examinations before coronary interventions, IVUS changed the treatment strategy by demonstrating more severe or milder coronary artery disease than appreciated by angiography. Also, IVUS remains an invaluable tool to evaluate adequate stent expansion or other suboptimal angiographic results.

Physiologic evaluation

Intracoronary Doppler

The coronary angiogram or IVUS offers no information regarding the coronary microcirculation, or of the physiologic significance of lesions. A physiologically significant lesion impairs coronary blood flow (CBF) at rest, or more commonly during stress [8,9].

At rest, myocardial demand is low, and accordingly CBF is at its lowest level. Under conditions of increased stimulation, the normal physiologic response to an increase in myocardial demand is enhanced CBF by vasodilation of epicardial and resistance vessels. The ability to increase CBF from resting CBF by reducing vasomotor tone to meet myocardial demand (hyperemia) is called coronary flow reserve (CFR). Normal individuals can increase CBF three- to fivefold to meet increased myocardial demand.

In the presence of a physiologically significant lesion, the resistance vessels compensate for the impaired CBF by vasodilating. In the case of a severe lesion, the resistance vessels are dilated fully. Thus, in response to a physiological or pharmacological stimulus that increases myocardial demand, the resistance vessels are not capable of further vasodilating, constituting a state of impaired CFR. Gould and Lipscomb demonstrated that the CFR is attenuated beginning with coronary artery stenosis of more than 50% of the diameter. Compensatory vasodilation of the distal coronary vascular bed maintains near normal resting flow for lesions between 70% and 85% of diameter stenosis, but adaptive vasodilation fails to compensate for lesions greater than 85% of diameter stenosis. These findings have served as reference for the current definition of obstructive coronary artery disease. Thus, it is accepted that at least 70% stenosis of an epicardial artery constitutes significantly obstructive coronary artery disease. It is clear, however, that lesions estimated to be 50% to 70% of diameter stenosis also may be physiologically significant, and hence may merit further evaluation. Using physiological assessments of intermediate lesions, it has been demonstrated that it is possible to safely defer an intervention in patients who have normal physiological parameters [10–12].

The CFR, defined as the ratio of hyperemic blood flow to resting blood flow, can be measured using a 0.014 inch intracoronary Doppler guide wire. CFR blood flow is calculated using the formula $\pi D^2 \times APV \div 8$, where D represents the coronary diameter measured 5 mm distal to the tip of the Doppler wire (by quantitative angiography or IVUS), and APV equals the average peak velocity from the Doppler tracing. The CFR is calculated by the ration of peak-to-baseline CBF in response to drug infusion or injection. When coronary artery diameter is presumed to remain unchanged in response to drug manipulation, the CFR is calculated by the ratio of peak-to-baseline flow velocity (APV). Normal value is greater than 2.5.

Common pharmacological drugs are used to detect abnormalities in CFR. Adenosine is thought to act on the coronary vasculature by stimulating the adenosine A2 receptor on smooth muscle cells. At high doses, adenosine can cross the endothelial barrier and stimulate the receptor on the smooth muscle directly in an endothelium-independent mechanism. Adenosine acts predominantly on vessels less than 150 μm in diameter, and, therefore, mainly assesses changes in the coronary resistance vessels as reflected by changes in coronary flow. The administration of adenosine provides mainly an endothelium-independent evaluation of the coronary microvasculature. Adenosine may cause bradyarrhythmias including sinus bradycardia and atrioventricular block, facial flushing, and bronchoconstriction. Because of the short half-life of adenosine, the duration of these effects is very brief.

It is important to recognize several possible pitfalls in the measurement of CFR using Doppler wire. Systemic conditions that may affect systemic hemodynamics such as thyrotoxicosis and anemia also may affect basal CFR. The microvasculature in infarcted areas of the myocardium may be impaired functionally. Caution should be exercised that the guidewire tip should not abut the vessel wall, should not be in a small branch, should not be distorted grossly in shape, and should not be placed in the proximity to a major bifurcation. In the left coronary artery system, the blood flow velocity in diastole is greater than in systole, perhaps because of the greater compression of the left ventricle during systole, whereas for the right coronary artery, the flow velocities are fairly similar during both phases. Although the basal CBF may be highest in the left anterior descending coronary artery and lowest in the right coronary artery, the CFR is fairly similar for all three major epicardial arteries. Because of the increased sensitivity of the right coronary artery to the pharmacological agents used, however, especially the chronotropic effects of adenosine, lower doses (18 to 24 μg) are recommended initially for injections to the right coronary artery, and doses of 30 to 40 μg are recommended for the left coronary system.

Coronary microvessels may have reduced vasodilating abilities because of structural or functional abnormalities (such as hypertension, diabetes mellitus), resulting in the ability to decrease vasomotor tone during stress. Therefore, in case of a low CFR ratio, CFR should be measured in another angiographically normal coronary artery. If the CFR is abnormally low in the control artery, diffuse coronary microvascular disease or another pathology should be sought (eg, diabetes mellitus or left ventricular hypertrophy). If the CFR in the control artery is normal, it is reasonable to assume that the lesion in question is physiologically significant.

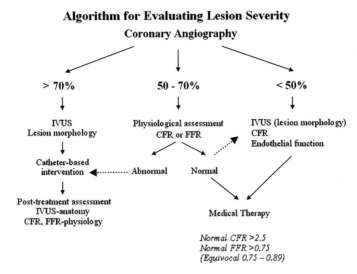

Fig. 3. Schematic flow chart to use anatomical and physiological lesion testing in decision-making process in the catheter laboratory.

Calculation of the relative CFR as the ratio of the CFR of the target lesion divided by the CFR of the normal vessel may be a more accurate assessment of the culprit lesion and generalized coronary microvasculature.

The use of CFR in cases with microvascular disease remains controversial. The inability of the microcirculation to respond to adenosine may result in inaccurate results. The ability of the Doppler wire to assess the microcirculation, however, may be considered an advantage in certain circumstances (ie, an impaired CFR measured in more than one epicardial artery may indicate coronary microvessel disease that may account for the patient's symptoms).

Fractional flow reserve

Fractional flow reserve (FFR) is a method for assessing indeterminate coronary artery stenoses based on pressure wire analysis during maximal flow. The concept of myocardial FFR, defined as the maximal blood flow to the myocardium in the presence of a stenosis in the supplying coronary artery, divided by the theoretical normal maximal flow in the same distribution, has been developed as an index of physiologic severity of the lesion. FFR represents the fraction of the normal maximal myocardial flow that can be achieved despite the coronary stenosis. This index can be calculated from the ratio of the mean distal coronary artery pressure to the aortic pressure during hyperemic maximal vasodilation. It is independent of changes in systemic blood pressure, heart rate, and status of microvascular circulation [13].

Moreover, the FFR takes into account the collateral blood supply. Per definition, the normal value of the FFR is 1.0 for any vessel investigated. Based on prior studies, it is accepted that an index value of less than 0.75 is abnormal and correlates well with pathological findings using noninvasive techniques. Appropriate interventions may reduce the future cardiac events. Values between 0.75 and 0.90 are of intermediate significance, and clinical correlation is suggested.

After calibration at zero, the wire is positioned distal to the lesion at question, and adenosine is administered (18 to 40 µg bolus) into the ostium of the coronary artery through the guiding catheter. The distal coronary pressure is monitored; maximal CBF is achieved with minimal coronary distal pressure. When the coronary distal pressure reaches a new steady state, the FFR is calculated by dividing the mean distal intracoronary pressure (measured by the pressure wire) by the mean arterial pressure (measured by the guiding catheter positioned in the ostium of the coronary artery).

Summary

Coronary angiography remains the gold standard of day-to-day lesion assessment. Other modalities may help to further improve the understanding of the lesion morphology for better management (Fig. 3).

References

[1] Ellis SG, Vandormael MG, Cowley MJ, et al. Coronary morphologic and clinical determinants of procedural outcome with angioplasty for multi-vessel coronary disease: implications for patient selection. Circulation 1990;82:1193–202.

[2] Ryan TJ, Faxon DP, Gunnar RM, et al. Guidelines for percutaneous transluminal coronary angioplasty: a report of the American College of Cardiology/American Heart Association Task Force on assessment of diagnostic and therapeutic cardiovascular procedures (subcommittee on percutaneous transluminal coronary angioplasty). J Am Coll Cardiol 1988;12:529–45.

[3] Krone RJ, Shaw RE, Klein LW, et al. Evaluation of the American College of Cardiology/American Heart Association and the Society for Coronary Angiography and Interventions lesion classification system in the current stent era of coronary interventions (from the ACC-National Cardiovascular Data Registry). Am J Cardiol 2003;92:389–94.

[4] Investigators EPISTENT. Randomised placebo-controlled and balloon angioplasty-controlled trial to assess safety of coronary stenting with use of platelet glycoprotein-IIb/IIIa blockade. Lancet 1998;352:87–92.

[5] Ellis SG, Guetta S, Miller D, et al. Relation between lesion characteristics and risk with percutaneous intervention in the stent and glycoprotein IIb/IIIa era—an analysis of results from 10 907 lesions and proposal for new classification scheme. Circulation 1999;100:1971–6.

[6] Saucedo JF, Lansjy AJ, Ito S, et al. A practical approach to quantitative coronary angiography. In: Beyar R, Keren G, Leon MB, et al, editors. Frontiers in interventional cardiology. London: Martin Dunitz Publishers; 1997. p. 281–96.

[7] Di Mario C, Gorge G, Peters R, et al. Clinical application and image interpretation in intracoronary ultrasound. Eur Heart J 1998;19:207–29.

[8] Pijls NH, de Bruyne B, Peels K, et al. Measurement of fractional flow reserve to assess the functional severity of coronary artery stenoses. N Engl J Med 1996;334:1703–8.

[9] Gould KL, Lipscomb K. Effects of coronary stenoses on coronary flow reserve and resistance. Am J Cardiol 1974;34:48–55.

[10] Kern M, Donohue T, Aguirre F, et al. Clinical outcome of deferring angioplasty in patients with normal translesional pressure flow velocity measurements. J Am Coll Cardiol 1995;25:178–87.

[11] Serruys P, di Mario C, Piek J, et al. Prognostic value of intracoronary flow velocity and diameter stenosis in assessing the short- and long-term outcomes of coronary balloon angioplasty: the DEBATE study (Doppler Endpoints Balloon Angioplasty Trial Europe). Circulation 1997;96:3369–77.

[12] Kern MJ, Meier B. Evaluation of the culprit plaque and the physiological significance of coronary atherosclerotic narrowings. Circulation 2001;103:3142–9.

[13] Pijls NH, de Bruyne B, Peels K, et al. Measurement of fractional flow reserve to assess the functional severity of coronary-artery stenoses. N Engl J Med 1996;334:1703–8.

ELSEVIER
SAUNDERS

Cardiol Clin 24 (2006) 163–173

CARDIOLOGY
CLINICS

Intravascular Ultrasound in the Current Percutaneous Coronary Intervention Era

Ilke Sipahi, MD[a], Stephen J. Nicholls, MBBS, PhD[b],
E. Murat Tuzcu, MD[a,c,*]

[a]Intravascular Ultrasound Core Laboratory, Department of Cardiovascular Medicine,
The Cleveland Clinic Foundation, 9500 Euclid Avenue, Desk JJ65, Cleveland, OH 44195, USA
[b]Interventional Cardiology, Department of Cardiovascular Medicine, The Cleveland Clinic Foundation,
9500 Euclid Avenue, Desk JJ65, Cleveland, OH 44195, USA
[c]Cleveland Clinic Lerner College of Medicine, Case Western Reserve University, 9500 Euclid Avenue,
Cleveland, OH 44195, USA

Intravascular ultrasound (IVUS) is an imaging modality that can bring a tomographic perspective to percutaneous coronary interventions (PCI). Although contrast angiography allows evaluation of lumen of coronary arteries in a planar fashion, it does not permit visualization of the arterial wall, which harbors the atherosclerotic tissue. IVUS is capable of showing the arterial wall and the lumen of the coronary arteries with high spatial resolution and across the full 360° circumference of the vessel. Thus, it provides additional information beyond what is obtained from angiography. The use of IVUS in the cardiac catheterization laboratory has continued to evolve since its introduction almost 15 years ago. In this review, the authors examine the role of IVUS in the current PCI era, which is dominated by the use of drug-eluting stents (DES).

Normal arterial anatomy and basic measurements by intravascular ultrasound

Normal coronary arteries usually have a tri-layered appearance on IVUS imaging, which corresponds to the three histologic layers of the arterial wall. The innermost layer is the echogenic intima, the middle layer is the echolucent media,

and outermost layer is the echogenic adventitia (Fig. 1). The upper limit of normal intimal thickness is considered to be 0.25 to 0.50 mm [1,2]. Lumen cross-sectional area (CSA) is determined by tracing the lumen–intima interface (Fig. 2). Minimum and maximum lumen diameters are the shortest and longest diameters through the center of the lumen. Because the outer border of adventitia is usually indistinct on IVUS imaging, total arterial CSA is measured by tracing the trailing edge of media and is referred to as external elastic membrane (EEM) CSA. Atheroma CSA is calculated as EEM CSA minus lumen CSA. Because atheroma CSA also includes the area occupied by the media, it is sometimes referred to as plaque plus media CSA. Atheroma CSA divided by EEM CSA yields percent CSA stenosis (or plaque burden). Percent CSA stenosis is distinct from percent diameter stenosis obtained by angiography because it is the fraction of arterial CSA occupied by atheroma at a single cross-section and does not use reference segments, unlike angiography. Detailed descriptions of standards of image acquisition and interpretation are available in the American College of Cardiology and the European Society of Cardiology expert consensus documents on IVUS [3,4].

Evaluation of intermediate coronary lesions

Making decisions for revascularization is a challenging task in patients who have intermediate

* Corresponding author. Department of Cardiovascular Medicine, The Cleveland Clinic Foundation, 9500 Euclid Avenue, Desk F25, Cleveland, OH 44195.
  E-mail address: tuzcue@ccf.org (E.M. Tuzcu).

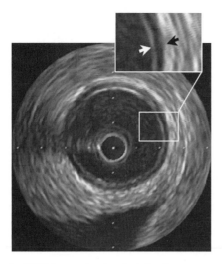

Fig. 1. IVUS image showing the trilaminar appearance of normal coronary arterial wall. White arrow points to the intima and black arrow points to the adventitia. The echolucent space between these two echogenic layers is the media. Note that all three layers may not be appreciable in some cases.

coronary lesions (ie, 40%–70% angiographic diameter stenosis). Intermediate lesions can be particularly troublesome in patients whose symptomatic status is difficult to evaluate. Vessel overlapping and tortuosity, lesion eccentricity, ostial localization, and severely calcified lesions can further compound the problem. In this context, IVUS is the alternative imaging modality and provides a tomographic perspective that often permits precise quantification of lumen and plaque

sizes. In addition, IVUS can help to assess the plaque morphology.

When an intermediate lesion is encountered, functional assessment using pressure or flow (Doppler) measurements is an important alternative to IVUS. Measurements of fractional flow reserve (FFR) and coronary flow reserve using miniaturized sensors have proved useful in identifying lesions of hemodynamic significance [5,6]. FFR data have been prospectively validated, and these studies have shown that deferring lesions with intermediate severity that are hemodynamically insignificant (ie, FFR>0.75) have favorable clinical follow-up [7]. The use of IVUS is preferred over functional studies when the anatomic distribution (eg, involvement of ostium or bifurcation) or the morphology of the lesion (eg, ulceration versus calcification as the cause of haziness on angiogram) is also important for decision-making. Unlike the case with functional studies, the accuracy of the IVUS cutoff values has not been validated prospectively by noninvasive tests of myocardial ischemia such as myocardial perfusion scintigraphy. Similarly, clinical outcome data for these cutoff values have been evaluated only in relatively small retrospective studies. The cutoff values for IVUS measurements that identify hemodynamically significant lesions have mostly been determined by correlating the lumen dimensions obtained during IVUS imaging with FFR and coronary flow reserve. A study of 51 lesions (not involving the left main coronary artery [LMCA]) found that a minimal lumen CSA of less than 3 mm^2 was the best cutoff value

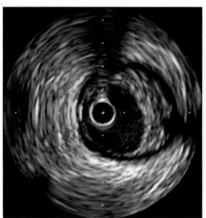
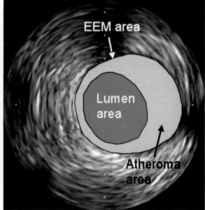

Fig. 2. IVUS image (*right panel*). Basic IVUS measurements (*left panel*). The area bound by the outer border of the echolucent media is the external elastic membrane (EEM) area. The area bound by the lumen-intima interface is the lumen area. EEM area minus lumen area yields the atheroma area.

for predicting hemodynamically significant lesions by FFR [8]. In a later study of 53 lesions, a minimal lumen CSA of less than 4 mm^2 and a minimal lumen diameter of less than 1.8 mm were found to be the best predictors of hemodynamic significance [9]. The apparent discrepancy between the cutoff values for minimal lumen CSA obtained in these two studies (3 versus 4 mm^2) may be due to the different agents used for inducing hyperemia (papaverine versus adenosine) or due to the very few number of lesions that had a minimal lumen CSA between 3 and 4 mm^2 in the former study. Because favorable clinical follow-up data are available for the minimum lumen area of 4.0 mm^2 [10], it is the authors' preference to use this parameter for decision making regarding revascularization for lesions that have intermediate severity. In the gray zone of 3 to 4 mm^2, the additional use of the criterion "percent CSA stenosis greater than 70%" [9] can be decisive because combining different criteria has been shown to increase specificity for hemodynamic significance [8]. It has been shown that a more precise evaluation of lesion severity using IVUS can change the decision about whether a lesion should be intervened in about 13% of the cases [11].

Evaluation of the left main coronary artery

It is often difficult to quantify the severity of LMCA stenoses by angiography [12,13]. Contrast in the aortic cusp can obscure the proximal part of the vessel, requiring the angiographer to engage the LMCA with the catheter and depend on the reflux of contrast to visualize the ostium. On the distal end, bifurcation or trifurcation into daughter branches may preclude accurate assessment. In some cases, the left main trunk is diffusely diseased, leaving no normal segment that can be used as a reference site. Because of these limitations, the reproducibility of quantitative coronary angiography (QCA) of the LMCA is worse than it is for the other coronary arterial segments [14,15]. When angiographic interpretation of the LMCA is uncertain, IVUS is usually a helpful modality because it does not suffer from the previously mentioned limitations of angiography (Fig. 3).

Certain technical issues should be considered when imaging the LMCA with IVUS. The IVUS probe should be placed in the straighter distal vessel (commonly the left anterior descending) and the guiding catheter should be disengaged to miss the ostium during the pullback. Selection of the guiding catheter is important to permit coaxial imaging. Short-tip JL-4 guiding catheters generally provide the ability to withdraw the tip while coaxiality is maintained.

Due to the larger caliber of the LMCA, criteria for the significance of LMCA lesions as assessed by IVUS are different from the rest of the coronary tree. In a study of 55 patients who had angiographically intermediate LMCA stenoses (49 $\pm$ 15% by QCA), a minimal luminal diameter of less than 2.8 mm and a minimal luminal CSA of less than 5.9 mm^2 were found to predict hemodynamically significant lesions with a sensitivity and specificity greater than 90% [16]. The cutoff value of 2.8 mm for minimal lumen diameter is also supported by a study with clinical end points [17]. This study, which included 122 patients who had intermediate stenoses in the LMCA (42 $\pm$ 16% by QCA), showed that minimal luminal diameter of the LMCA as measured by IVUS was the strongest predictor of cardiac events during the 1-year follow-up. In this study, a minimal luminal diameter of 3 mm performed best as a threshold value and, accordingly, patients who had a minimal lumen diameter greater than 3 mm had an event rate of only 3%. A recent study that also used clinical end points has suggested that a minimal lumen CSA of 7.5 mm^2, a value higher than the 5.9 mm^2 dictated by the FFR study, should be used as the cutoff value for performing revascularization [18]. This value, however, was obtained not according to event rates but by calculating the mean minus 2 SD of minimal lumen areas in a group of patients who had completely normal LMCAs. As a result, it is the authors' preference to use the criterion "minimal lumen diameter less than 2.8 mm" for revascularization in LMCA lesions, which has been validated by clinical end point and functional studies.

Intravascular ultrasound for guidance of stenting

IVUS imaging has been instrumental in understanding the arterial responses to almost every single interventional modality and has helped to improve the technical details about the manufacturing and the use of most of the coronary devices. Despite its profound impact on the refinement of various percutaneous coronary procedures, it should be noted that routine IVUS guidance for coronary interventions, particularly while using DES, is not a requirement.

IVUS imaging has played a pivotal role, especially in optimizing the technique of stent deployment as it is currently practiced. IVUS

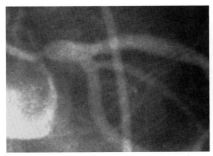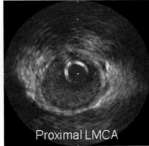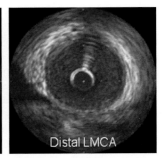

Proximal LMCA   Distal LMCA

Fig. 3. Coronary angiogram (*left panel*) shows severe stenosis of the LMCA ostium; however, IVUS reveals that the left main stem has no atherosclerotic disease (*middle and right panels*). On the other hand, the lumen of the proximal vessel is smaller than that of the distal vessel, which is the reason of the angiographic appearance. This phenomenon is referred to as "reverse tapering."

observations revealed that the earlier technique of coronary stenting used in the initial randomized stent trials frequently resulted in incomplete expansion and imperfect apposition of the stent struts, despite the satisfactory angiographic results [19,20]. These observations led to critical refinements in the technique of stenting, which included higher-pressure postdilations and the use of larger-sized balloons. These developments, together with the use of dual antiplatelet therapy, substantially reduced the incidence of subacute stent thrombosis [21], and the use of oral anticoagulation was no longer needed.

After the observation of the adverse consequences of underexpanded and unapposed stents, which included stent thrombosis and restenosis, the possible benefits of IVUS-guided stenting over angiography-guided stenting were evaluated vigorously in several nonrandomized registries [22–26], randomized trials [27–29], and in a meta-analysis of these data sources [30]. The incidence of death or myocardial infarction was not altered by IVUS guidance in any of these studies. In the registries, IVUS guidance generally reduced the angiographic binary restenosis and target vessel revascularization rates, probably by promoting larger postprocedural minimal lumen CSAs. However, randomized trials produced mixed results. In the relatively small Restenosis After IVUS-Guided Stenting (RESIST) trial, there was a nonsignificant reduction in the angiographic binary restenosis rate in the IVUS-guided arm (28.8% to 22.5%, $P = 0.25$) [27]. Optimization with ICUS to reduce stent restinosis (OPTICUS), the largest reported randomized trial on the comparison of IVUS-guided versus angiography-guided stenting, specifically included lesions 25 mm or less in length that had a 2.5 mm or

greater reference segment diameter. Results of OPTICUS showed similar restenosis rates (24.5% versus 22.8%, $P = 0.68$) and similar target vessel revascularization rates in the two arms [28]. The thrombocyte activity evaluation and effects of ultrasound guidance in long coronary stent replacement (TULIP) Study [29] investigated the role of IVUS in stenting diffuse (≥ 20 mm) coronary lesions. In this study, the restenosis rate was lower with IVUS guidance (46% versus 23%, $P = 0.008$), as was the target lesion revascularization rate (14% versus 4%, $P = 0.037$). Postintervention minimal lumen diameter, the number of stents used in each patient, average stent length, and final balloon size were all greater in the IVUS-guided group. The positive impact of IVUS guidance in TULIP, as opposed to the neutral results of OPTICUS, implies that IVUS guidance can reduce restenosis in patients who are at a particularly high risk for restenosis. Various criteria have been suggested for optimal stent expansion using IVUS-guidance [31–33]. For implanting a bare metal stent, the criteria "minimal stent CSA greater than 7 mm^2" and "minimal lumen CSA divided by reference EEM CSA greater than 0.55" are probably the most useful (Fig. 4) [33].

With DES, the frequency of restenosis has been reduced to less than 10% [34,35]. Therefore, with the more widespread use of DES, the potential advantage of IVUS guidance to reduce restenosis is less significant. Stent underexpansion, however, may still be a major cause of restenosis with DES. Two studies have shown that with sirolimus-eluting stents, a postprocedural minimum stent area of less than 5 mm^2 was a strong predictor of angiographic binary restenosis or a follow-up minimal lumen area of less than 4 mm^2 [36,37],

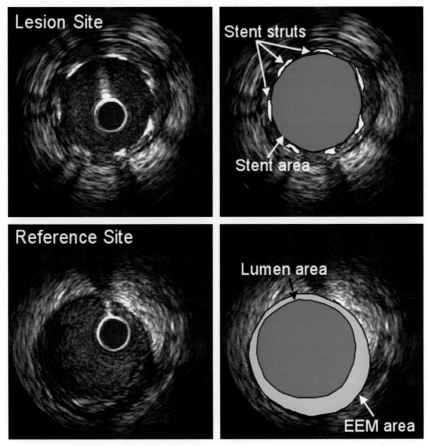

Fig. 4. Example of a well-expanded stent (*upper panels*). The stent area is 8.0 mm^2. The reference lumen area is 9.3 mm^2 and reference EEM area is 13.5 mm^2 (*lower panels*). These measurements show that this is a well-expanded stent by most criteria. Note the complete apposition of the stent struts to the arterial wall.

which is an indicator of a hemodynamically significant lesion [9]. In addition to its association with restenosis, stent underexpansion has been associated with stent thrombosis in DES [38]; thus, it is thought that in selected patients, higher inflation pressures (>18 atm) may be needed to achieve a minimum acceptable stent CSA and, therefore, to prevent restenosis and thrombosis in DES [37]. Although routine IVUS guidance for better expansion of DES is probably not feasible, IVUS examination may be warranted when it is difficult to choose the diameter of the stent to be placed (eg, when there is a large difference in the diameters of the proximal and the distal reference segments or when the artery is diffusely diseased). Although there is no firm guideline to determine the stent size to be placed in a diffusely diseased artery using IVUS imaging, one can use the method followed in the Clinical Outcomes with

Ultrasound Trial (CLOUT) in which IVUS was used for balloon sizing [39]. Accordingly, if a "normal" reference diameter is not available, one can estimate the stent diameter to be the average of the lumen and EEM diameters at the least diseased site. In addition, stent length is particularly important when a DES is used because in addition to stent underexpansion, residual proximal or distal segment stenosis on IVUS imaging has been associated with stent thrombosis [37]. Therefore, it is important to cover the entire diseased area. IVUS is also useful for stent positioning when the degree of osteal involvement cannot be discerned by angiography. In such situations, IVUS can reliably determine whether the "true ostium" is diseased, in which case the stent should cover the ostium and can actually protrude into the parent branch. In other cases in which a few millimeters of the most proximal portion of the target vessel harbors no disease, the stent can be anchored to the most proximal disease-free segment.

In the past, IVUS has been used to evaluate morphology of the lesions in an effort to optimize selection of interventional devices (ie, rotational atherectomy for heavily calcified lesions versus directional atherectomy for others). With the predominance of stenting, and particularly of DES, evidence supporting the use of IVUS imaging to aid in PCI device selection has become obsolete. IVUS, however, can still be helpful in cases of directional coronary atherectomy because angiography is sometimes incapable of localizing the tissue for retrieval, especially in eccentric lesions.

Assessing complications of intervention using intravascular ultrasound

Coronary dissection is the most common reason for acute arterial closure during PCI and can result in serious complications including death, myocardial infarction, and emergent bypass surgery. In addition, residual dissection after stenting remains a risk factor for subacute stent thrombosis in the DES era [40]. For detection of dissections, IVUS is a much more sensitive imaging modality than angiography. The circumferential and the longitudinal extent of coronary dissections can be better appreciated by IVUS (Fig. 5). Because IVUS has not been shown to improve outcomes when evaluating coronary dissections, interventionalists prefer to assess this condition by angiography alone. Most nonflow limiting dissections that have no high-risk features

on angiography (ie, extraluminal dye staining, filling defects, or spiral dissections) can be treated conservatively without additional mechanical interventions. Whenever there is an indication for stenting, IVUS imaging usually reveals involvement of a longer arterial segment than can be appreciated angiographically. This additional involvement may be particularly important in cases of bailout stenting for threatened acute closure, in which it is critical to cover the entirety of the dissected segment. In such cases, presence of a residual dissection in the vicinity of the bailout stent or stents adds to the already higher risk of stent thrombosis [41]. Residual dissection also remains a risk factor for subacute stent thrombosis in the DES era [40], although the absolute risk of thrombosis seems to be low.

"Peristent haziness" is used to refer to the nonhomogenous density or ground-glass appearance on the angiogram that generally occurs proximal or distal to the stented segment. In some cases of peristent haziness, an obvious cause (eg, a dissection or a thrombus) can readily be seen on angiograms. In others, there is no obvious cause, and such persistent haziness has been reported to be 15% with high-pressure stenting. In these types of cases in which the etiology cannot be readily appreciated by angiogram, IVUS imaging can be helpful. With IVUS, major causes of this phenomenon have been found to be dissections, significant step-down of luminal area from the edge of the stent to a segment of moderate disease [42], and calcifications without any dissections [43]. In the cases of calcification or luminal step-down as the cause of persistent haziness, IVUS imaging can prevent

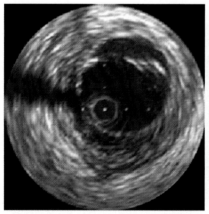 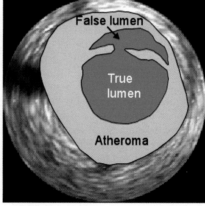

Fig. 5. IVUS image (*left panel*). Example of a coronary dissection occurring after balloon dilatation (*right panel*). The intimal tear at the 12-o'clock position connects the true lumen with the false lumen.

Box 1. American College of Cardiology/American Heart Association recommendations for coronary intravascular ultrasound

Class I
None
Class IIa
1. Assessment of the adequacy of deployment of coronary stents, including the extent of stent apposition and determination of the minimum luminal diameter within the stent. (Level of evidence: B)
2. Determination of the mechanism of stent restenosis (inadequate expansion versus neointimal proliferation) and to enable selection of appropriate therapy (plaque ablation versus repeat balloon expansion). (Level of evidence: B)
3. Evaluation of coronary obstruction at a location difficult to image by angiography in a patient with a suspected flow-limiting stenosis. (Level of evidence: C)
4. Assessment of a suboptimal angiographic result following PCI. (Level of evidence: C)
5. Diagnosis and management of coronary disease following cardiac transplantation. (Level of evidence: C)
6. Establish presence and distribution of coronary calcium in patients for whom adjunctive rotational atherectomy is contemplated. (Level of evidence: C)
7. Determination of plaque location and circumferential distribution for guidance of directional coronary atherectomy. (Level of evidence: B)
Class IIb
1. Determine extent of atherosclerosis in patients with characteristic anginal symptoms and a positive functional study with no focal stenoses or mild coronary artery disease on angiography. (Level of evidence: C)
2. Preinterventional assessment of lesional characteristics and vessel dimensions as a means to select an optimal revascularization device. (Level of evidence: C)
Class III
1. When angiographic diagnosis is clear and no interventional treatment is planned. (Level of evidence: C)
This document employs the American College of Cardiology/American Heart Association style classification of class I, II, or III. These classes summarize the indications for PCI as follows:
Class I—conditions for which there is evidence for and/or general agreement that the procedure or treatment is useful and effective
Class II—conditions for which there is conflicting evidence and/or a divergence of opinion about the usefulness/efficacy of a procedure or treatment
Class IIa—weight of evidence/opinion is in favor of usefulness/efficacy
Class IIb—usefulness/efficacy is less well established by evidence/opinion
Class III—conditions for which there is evidence and/or general agreement that the procedure/treatment is not useful/effective and, in some cases, may be harmful.
The weight of evidence in support of the recommendation for each listed indication is presented as follows:
Level of evidence A—data derived from multiple randomized clinical trials
Level of evidence B—data derived from a single randomized trial or nonrandomized studies
Level of evidence C—consensus opinion of experts

From Smith SC Jr, Dove JT, Jacobs AK, et al. ACC/AHA guidelines for percutaneous coronary intervention (revision of the 1993 PTCA guidelines)—executive summary: a report of the American College of Cardiology/American Heart Association task force on practice guidelines (Committee to Revise the 1993 Guidelines for Percutaneous Transluminal Coronary Angioplasty) endorsed by the Society for Cardiac Angiography and Interventions. Circulation 2001;103(24):3019–41.

unnecessary deployment of additional stents and, therefore, may reduce the risk of restenosis and the cost of the procedure.

Intravascular ultrasound for the management of stent restenosis

Despite advances in the technique of stent deployment, adjuvant pharmacologic therapies, and the use of DES that inhibit neointimal proliferation, stent restenosis remains a problem of interventional cardiology.

IVUS has provided substantial insight into the mechanisms of stent restenosis [44–46]. Using IVUS, it was found that about 20% of bare metal stent restenosis cases harbor unexpanded stents [47,48]. The relative contribution of stent underexpansion is even greater in cases of DES restenosis [37,49,50].

The authors believe that IVUS should be used in decision making for the treatment of stent restenosis. If IVUS identifies stent underexpansion as the cause of restenosis site, balloon dilatations based on IVUS stent area measurements should be the mode of treatment. If neointimal proliferation is found to be the cause, then restenting should be considered. The exact localization of the restenotic site is also important when deciding among treatment options. If restenosis is within the stent, then higher-pressure inflations can be effective. Conversely, this approach may not be suitable for treating "edge restenosis" that occurs in the unstented nearby reference sites.

In the DES era, the binary restenosis rate is low and, therefore, in clinical studies large numbers of patients are needed to have enough power to detect a difference in the efficacy of different DES. In-stent late lumen loss, as determined by IVUS, has been used by some investigators to compare the efficacy of various strategies including different DES or the long-term results in different patient populations [51]. It is currently unknown whether a larger late loss as determined by IVUS is associated with significantly higher clinical event rates.

Guidelines

The latest recommendations of the American College of Cardiology and the American Heart Association on indications for coronary IVUS are published in the 2001 guidelines for PCI [52]. Box 1 summarizes these recommendations. The results of recent research presented in this review and the declining use of most of the interventional devices other than DES are likely to change some of these recommendations.

Identification of vulnerable plaques: the future of intravascular ultrasound imaging?

Currently, decisions regarding the percutaneous treatment of coronary lesions are mostly driven by the degree of luminal compromise as assessed by the angiogram or by complementary studies such as pressure measurements or IVUS.

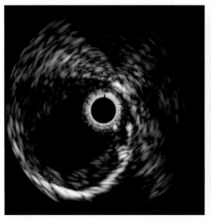 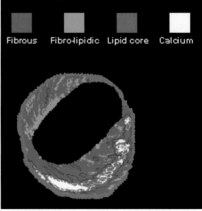

Fig. 6. Left panel shows a regular gray-scale IVUS image of an atherosclerotic plaque. Right panel shows tissue characterization map obtained through spectral analysis of the same cross-section.

Accurate identification of plaques that do not cause significant luminal compromise but are vulnerable to future rupture can revolutionize not only the percutaneous but also the pharmacologic treatment of coronary artery disease. Although regular gray-scale IVUS can help to estimate various histologic components of plaques, particularly calcifications, it cannot reliably differentiate vulnerable plaques from stable plaques. Accordingly, various techniques based on IVUS imaging (elastography, palpography, spectral analysis) or other imaging modalities (optical coherence tomography, thermography, intracoronary magnetic resonance) have been developed for detection of vulnerable plaques [53]. Of the IVUS-based modalities, IVUS elastography evaluates the local elastic properties (strain) of plaques and has been shown to detect histologically vulnerable plaques with high sensitivity and specificity [54]. IVUS palpography is an allied technology that also evaluates tissue strain but is faster and more robust than IVUS elastography [55]. Spectral analysis of radiofrequency signals is another promising new IVUS-based imaging modality. This technique has been shown to classify various components of plaques with high accuracy (Fig. 6) [56,57] and has been used successfully to evaluate changes in these components with lipid-lowering therapy [58]. Ongoing research including the Providing Regional Observations to Study Predictors of Events in the Coronary Tree (PROSPECT) study will help define the value of radiofrequency spectral analysis and other novel coronary imaging modalities in determining or improving clinical outcomes.

References

[1] St. Goar FG, Pinto FJ, Alderman EL, et al. Intravascular ultrasound imaging of angiographically normal coronary arteries: an in vivo comparison with quantitative angiography. J Am Coll Cardiol 1991;18(4):952–8.

[2] Fitzgerald PJ, St. Goar FG, Connolly AJ, et al. Intravascular ultrasound imaging of coronary arteries. Is three layers the norm? Circulation 1992;86(1):154–8.

[3] Mintz GS, Nissen SE, Anderson WD, et al. American College of Cardiology Clinical Expert Consensus Document on Standards for Acquisition, Measurement and Reporting of Intravascular Ultrasound Studies (IVUS). A report of the American College of Cardiology Task Force on Clinical Expert Consensus Documents. J Am Coll Cardiol 2001; 37(5):1478–92.

[4] Di Mario C, Gorge G, Peters R, et al. Clinical application and image interpretation in intracoronary ultrasound. Study group on Intracoronary Imaging of the Working Group of Coronary Circulation and of the Subgroup on Intravascular Ultrasound of the Working Group of Echocardiography of the European Society of Cardiology. Eur Heart J 1998; 19(2):207–29.

[5] Pijls NH, De Bruyne B, Peels K, et al. Measurement of fractional flow reserve to assess the functional severity of coronary-artery stenoses. N Engl J Med 1996;334(26):1703–8.

[6] Miller DD, Donohue TJ, Younis LT, et al. Correlation of pharmacological 99mTc-sestamibi myocardial perfusion imaging with poststenotic coronary flow reserve in patients with angiographically intermediate coronary artery stenoses. Circulation 1994; 89(5):2150–60.

[7] Bech GJ, De Bruyne B, Pijls NH, et al. Fractional flow reserve to determine the appropriateness of angioplasty in moderate coronary stenosis: a randomized trial. Circulation 2001;103(24):2928–34.

[8] Takagi A, Tsurumi Y, Ishii Y, et al. Clinical potential of intravascular ultrasound for physiological assessment of coronary stenosis: relationship between quantitative ultrasound tomography and pressure-derived fractional flow reserve. Circulation 1999; 100(3):250–5.

[9] Briguori C, Anzuini A, Airoldi F, et al. Intravascular ultrasound criteria for the assessment of the functional significance of intermediate coronary artery stenoses and comparison with fractional flow reserve. Am J Cardiol 2001;87(2):136–41.

[10] Abizaid AS, Mintz GS, Mehran R, et al. Long-term follow-up after percutaneous transluminal coronary angioplasty was not performed based on intravascular ultrasound findings: importance of lumen dimensions. Circulation 1999;100(3):256–61.

[11] Mintz GS, Pichard AD, Kovach JA, et al. Impact of preintervention intravascular ultrasound imaging on transcatheter treatment strategies in coronary artery disease. Am J Cardiol 1994;73(7): 423–30.

[12] Isner JM, Kishel J, Kent KM, et al. Accuracy of angiographic determination of left main coronary arterial narrowing. Angiographic-histologic correlative analysis in 28 patients. Circulation 1981;63(5): 1056–64.

[13] Cameron A, Kemp HG Jr, Fisher LD, et al. Left main coronary artery stenosis: angiographic determination. Circulation 1983;68(3):484–9.

[14] Prospective randomised study of coronary artery bypass surgery in stable angina pectoris. Second interim report by the European Coronary Surgery Study Group. Lancet 1980;2(8193):491–5.

[15] Fisher LD, Judkins MP, Lesperance J, et al. Reproducibility of coronary arteriographic reading in the coronary artery surgery study (CASS). Cathet Cardiovasc Diagn 1982;8(6):565–75.

[16] Jasti V, Ivan E, Yalamanchili V, et al. Correlations between fractional flow reserve and intravascular ultrasound in patients with an ambiguous left main coronary artery stenosis. Circulation 2004;110(18): 2831–6.

[17] Abizaid AS, Mintz GS, Abizaid A, et al. One-year follow-up after intravascular ultrasound assessment of moderate left main coronary artery disease in patients with ambiguous angiograms. J Am Coll Cardiol 1999;34(3):707–15.

[18] Fassa AA, Wagatsuma K, Higano ST, et al. Intravascular ultrasound-guided treatment for angiographically indeterminate left main coronary artery disease: a long-term follow-up study. J Am Coll Cardiol 2005;45(2):204–11.

[19] Nakamura S, Colombo A, Gaglione A, et al. Intracoronary ultrasound observations during stent implantation. Circulation 1994;89(5):2026–34.

[20] Kiemeneij F, Laarman G, Slagboom T. Mode of deployment of coronary Palmaz-Schatz stents after implantation with the stent delivery system: an intravascular ultrasound study. Am Heart J 1995; 129(4):638–44.

[21] Colombo A, Hall P, Nakamura S, et al. Intracoronary stenting without anticoagulation accomplished with intravascular ultrasound guidance. Circulation 1995;91(6):1676–88.

[22] Albiero R, Rau T, Schluter M, et al. Comparison of immediate and intermediate-term results of intravascular ultrasound versus angiography-guided Palmaz-Schatz stent implantation in matched lesions. Circulation 1997;96(9):2997–3005.

[23] Blasini R, Neumann FJ, Schmitt C, et al. Restenosis rate after intravascular ultrasound-guided coronary stent implantation. Cathet Cardiovasc Diagn 1998; 44(4):380–6.

[24] Fitzgerald PJ, Oshima A, Hayase M, et al. Final results of the Can Routine Ultrasound Influence Stent Expansion (CRUISE) study. Circulation 2000; 102(5):523–30.

[25] Choi JW, Goodreau LM, Davidson CJ. Resource utilization and clinical outcomes of coronary stenting: a comparison of intravascular ultrasound and angiographical guided stent implantation. Am Heart J 2001;142(1):112–8.

[26] Orford JL, Denktas AE, Williams BA, et al. Routine intravascular ultrasound scanning guidance of coronary stenting is not associated with improved clinical outcomes. Am Heart J 2004;148(3):501–6.

[27] Schiele F, Meneveau N, Vuillemenot A, et al. Impact of intravascular ultrasound guidance in stent deployment on 6-month restenosis rate: a multicenter, randomized study comparing two strategies—with and without intravascular ultrasound guidance. RESIST Study Group. REStenosis after Ivus guided STenting. J Am Coll Cardiol 1998;32(2): 320–8.

[28] Mudra H, di Mario C, de Jaegere P, et al. Randomized comparison of coronary stent implantation under ultrasound or angiographic guidance to reduce stent restenosis (OPTICUS Study). Circulation 2001;104(12):1343–9.

[29] Oemrawsingh PV, Mintz GS, Schalij MJ, et al. Intravascular ultrasound guidance improves angiographic and clinical outcome of stent implantation for long coronary artery stenoses: final results of a randomized comparison with angiographic guidance (TULIP Study). Circulation 2003;107(1):62–7.

[30] Casella G, Klauss V, Ottani F, et al. Impact of intravascular ultrasound-guided stenting on long-term clinical outcome: a meta-analysis of available studies comparing intravascular ultrasound-guided and angiographically guided stenting. Catheter Cardiovasc Interv 2003;59(3):314–21.

[31] Hoffmann R, Mintz GS, Mehran R, et al. Intravascular ultrasound predictors of angiographic restenosis in lesions treated with Palmaz-Schatz stents. J Am Coll Cardiol 1998;31(1):43–9.

[32] de Jaegere P, Mudra H, Figulla H, et al. Intravascular ultrasound-guided optimized stent deployment. Immediate and 6 months clinical and angiographic results from the Multicenter Ultrasound Stenting in Coronaries Study (MUSIC Study). Eur Heart J 1998;19(8):1214–23.

[33] Moussa I, Moses J, Di Mario C, et al. Does the specific intravascular ultrasound criterion used to optimize stent expansion have an impact on the probability of stent restenosis? Am J Cardiol 1999; 83(7):1012–7.

[34] Moses JW, Leon MB, Popma JJ, et al. Sirolimus-eluting stents versus standard stents in patients with stenosis in a native coronary artery. N Engl J Med 2003;349(14):1315–23.

[35] Schofer J, Schluter M, Gershlick AH, et al. Sirolimus-eluting stents for treatment of patients with long atherosclerotic lesions in small coronary arteries: double-blind, randomised controlled trial (E-SIRIUS). Lancet 2003;362(9390):1093–9.

[36] Sonoda S, Morino Y, Ako J, et al. Impact of final stent dimensions on long-term results following sirolimus-eluting stent implantation: serial intravascular ultrasound analysis from the SIRIUS trial. J Am Coll Cardiol 2004;43(11):1959–63.

[37] Fujii K, Mintz GS, Kobayashi Y, et al. Contribution of stent underexpansion to recurrence after sirolimus-eluting stent implantation for in-stent restenosis. Circulation 2004;109(9):1085–8.

[38] Fujii K, Carlier SG, Mintz GS, et al. Stent underexpansion and residual reference segment stenosis are related to stent thrombosis after sirolimus-eluting stent implantation: an intravascular ultrasound study. J Am Coll Cardiol 2005;45(7):995–8.

[39] Stone GW, Hodgson JM, St. Goar FG, et al. Improved procedural results of coronary angioplasty with intravascular ultrasound-guided balloon sizing: the CLOUT Pilot Trial. Clinical Outcomes with Ultrasound Trial (CLOUT) Investigators. Circulation 1997;95(8):2044–52.

[40] Regar E, Lemos PA, Saia F, et al. Incidence of thrombotic stent occlusion during the first three months after sirolimus-eluting stent implantation in 500 consecutive patients. Am J Cardiol 2004; 93(10):1271–5.

[41] Schuhlen H, Hadamitzky M, Walter H, et al. Major benefit from antiplatelet therapy for patients at high risk for adverse cardiac events after coronary Palmaz-Schatz stent placement: analysis of a prospective risk stratification protocol in the Intracoronary Stenting and Antithrombotic Regimen (ISAR) trial. Circulation 1997;95(8):2015–21.

[42] Ziada KM, Tuzcu EM, De Franco AC, et al. Intravascular ultrasound assessment of the prevalence and causes of angiographic "haziness" following high-pressure coronary stenting. Am J Cardiol 1997;80(2):116–21.

[43] Grewal J, Ganz P, Selwyn A, et al. Usefulness of intravascular ultrasound in preventing stenting of hazy areas adjacent to coronary stents and its support of support spot-stenting. Am J Cardiol 2001; 87(11):1246–9.

[44] Painter JA, Mintz GS, Wong SC, et al. Serial intravascular ultrasound studies fail to show evidence of chronic Palmaz-Schatz stent recoil. Am J Cardiol 1995;75(5):398–400.

[45] Hoffmann R, Mintz GS, Dussaillant GR, et al. Patterns and mechanisms of in-stent restenosis. A serial intravascular ultrasound study. Circulation 1996; 94(6):1247–54.

[46] Lemos PA, Saia F, Ligthart JM, et al. Coronary restenosis after sirolimus-eluting stent implantation: morphological description and mechanistic analysis from a consecutive series of cases. Circulation 2003; 108(3):257–60.

[47] Castagna MT, Mintz GS, Leiboff BO, et al. The contribution of "mechanical" problems to in-stent restenosis: an intravascular ultrasonographic analysis of 1090 consecutive in-stent restenosis lesions. Am Heart J 2001;142(6):970–4.

[48] Sharma SK, Kini A, Mehran R, et al. Randomized trial of Rotational Atherectomy Versus Balloon Angioplasty for Diffuse In-stent Restenosis (ROSTER). Am Heart J 2004;147(1):16–22.

[49] Takebayashi H, Kobayashi Y, Mintz GS, et al. Intravascular ultrasound assessment of lesions with target vessel failure after sirolimus-eluting stent implantation. Am J Cardiol 2005;95(4):498–502.

[50] Cheneau E, Pichard AD, Satler LF, et al. Intravascular ultrasound stent area of sirolimus-eluting stents and its impact on late outcome. Am J Cardiol 2005;95(10):1240–2.

[51] Abizaid A, Costa MA, Blanchard D, et al. Sirolimus-eluting stents inhibit neointimal hyperplasia in diabetic patients. Insights from the RAVEL Trial. Eur Heart J 2004;25(2):107–12.

[52] Smith SC Jr, Dove JT, Jacobs AK, et al. ACC/AHA guidelines for percutaneous coronary intervention (revision of the 1993 PTCA guidelines)—executive summary: a report of the American College of Cardiology/American Heart Association task force on practice guidelines (Committee to Revise the 1993 Guidelines for Percutaneous Transluminal Coronary Angioplasty) endorsed by the Society for Cardiac Angiography and Interventions. Circulation 2001;103(24):3019–41.

[53] Tuzcu EM, Schoenhagen P. Acute coronary syndromes, plaque vulnerability, and carotid artery disease: the changing role of atherosclerosis imaging. J Am Coll Cardiol 2003;42(6):1033–6.

[54] Schaar JA, De Korte CL, Mastik F, et al. Characterizing vulnerable plaque features with intravascular elastography. Circulation 2003;108(21):2636–41.

[55] Schaar JA, Regar E, Mastik F, et al. Incidence of high-strain patterns in human coronary arteries: assessment with three-dimensional intravascular palpography and correlation with clinical presentation. Circulation 2004;109(22):2716–9.

[56] Nair A, Kuban BD, Tuzcu EM, et al. Coronary plaque classification with intravascular ultrasound radiofrequency data analysis. Circulation 2002; 106(17):2200–6.

[57] Murashige A, Hiro T, Fujii T, et al. Detection of lipid-laden atherosclerotic plaque by wavelet analysis of radiofrequency intravascular ultrasound signals: in vitro validation and preliminary in vivo application. J Am Coll Cardiol 2005;45(12):1954–60.

[58] Kawasaki M, Sano K, Okubo M, et al. Volumetric quantitative analysis of tissue characteristics of coronary plaques after statin therapy using three-dimensional integrated backscatter intravascular ultrasound. J Am Coll Cardiol 2005;45(12):1946–53.

**ELSEVIER
SAUNDERS**

Cardiol Clin 24 (2006) 175–199

**CARDIOLOGY
CLINICS**

Antithrombotic Therapy for Percutaneous Coronary Intervention

Nitin Barman, MD[a], Deepak L. Bhatt, MD[b],*

[a]*Interventional Cardiology, Mount Sinai Hospital, One Gustave L. Levy Place, New York, NY 10029, USA*
[b]*Cardiac, Peripheral, and Carotid Intervention, Department of Cardiovascular Medicine,
Cleveland Clinic Foundation, 9500 Euclid Avenue, Desk F25, Cleveland, OH 44195, USA*

The use of percutaneous coronary intervention (PCI) in the treatment of obstructive coronary artery disease has expanded rapidly in the past decade. Despite extensive technologic advancements in the field, pharmacotherapy has remained a cornerstone in the overall treatment strategy. Optimizing the ischemic complications mediated through a complex coagulation cascade, with the ever-present risk of bleeding from antiplatelet and anticoagulant therapy, has a remained a challenge for drug developers and for clinicians. In this article, the authors discuss the evolution, current treatment, and future landscape of pharmacotherapy in PCI.

Platelet biology

Comprehension of platelet biology has provided the basis for the current standard of antiplatelet therapy in PCI. Circulating platelets traverse the vasculature in an inactivated state until they are exposed to collagen fibrils in the connective tissue matrix underlying normal endothelial cells. Exposure to this matrix, which occurs universally after vessel injury induced by PCI, results in a complex series of events leading to platelet activation and aggregation. Activated platelets change their configuration and secrete, among other substances, thromboxane A_2 and ADP into the local environment, resulting in amplification of circulating platelet activation. Parallel pathways of platelet activation exist, including the interaction of tissue factor (TF), which is expressed on all nonvascular cells, and factor VIIa. This interaction results in the generation of thrombin, the most potent of platelet activators, and local coagulation. The final pathway of aggregation of platelets, which leads to the platelet thrombus, is mediated through the glycoprotein IIb/IIIa receptor. Activated platelets allow for conformational changes and upregulation of surface expression of the IIb/IIIa receptor. These conformation changes allow for fibrinogen binding and cross-linking of platelets, with the ultimate result being growth and stability of the hemostatic plug (Fig. 1). Because initial platelet thrombus formation during PCI plays a major role in acute and subacute periprocedural ischemic complications, it is no surprise that this pathway has been a major target for pharmacotherapy in PCI.

Antiplatelet agents

Aspirin

The use of aspirin is ubiquitous in patients undergoing coronary intervention. By acetylating the cyclooxygenase-1 enzyme, aspirin inhibits the synthesis of thromboxane A_2, resulting in irreversible inhibition of platelet function. Daily administration of 30 to 50 mg of aspirin results in virtually complete suppression of thromboxane A_2 synthesis by 7 to 10 days [1,2]. Justification for the use of aspirin in PCI is based primarily on a number of early trials that compared aspirin and dipyridamole versus placebo before percutaneous transluminal coronary angioplasty (PTCA). These studies demonstrated a statistically significant

---

* Corresponding author.
E-mail address: bhattd@ccf.org (D.L. Bhatt).

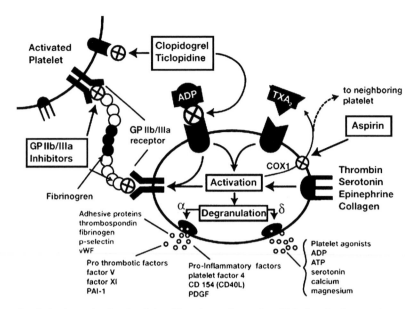

Fig. 1. Schematic of platelet activation involving (1) a shape change in which the platelet membrane surface area is greatly increased; (2) the secretion of proinflammatory, prothrombotic, adhesive, and chemotactic mediators that propagate, amplify, and sustain the atherothrombotic process; and (3) the activation of the glycoprotein (GP) IIb/IIIa receptor from its inactive form. Multiple agonists including thromboxane A_2 (TXA$_2$), ADP, thrombin, serotonin, epinephrine, and collagen can activate the platelet and, thus, contribute toward establishing the environmental conditions necessary for atherothrombosis to occur. COX1, cyclooxygenase-1; PAI, plasminogen activator inhibitor; PDGF, platelet-derived growth factor; vWF, von Willebrand factor. (*From* Mehta SR, Yusuf S. Short- and long-term oral antiplatelet therapy in acute coronary syndromes and percutaneous coronary intervention. J Am Coll Cardiol 2003;41(4):S79–88; with permission.)

reduction in periprocedural ischemic complications including abrupt vessel closure, Q wave myocardial infarction (MI), or need for emergent coronary artery bypass grafting (5% versus 14%) [3,4]. Further study demonstrated that these benefits were present irrespective of the use of dipyrimadole, which has subsequently fallen out of favor in the treatment of patients undergoing PCI [5]. With respect to dose, the initial trials of aspirin all used high doses of aspirin (> 650 mg/d), although subsequent study has suggested an absence of additional efficacy beyond 81 mg/d used chronically [6,7]. Due to the higher dose of aspirin used initially after PCI in more recent randomized studies, current recommendations are for 325 mg daily for 1 month following bare metal stent or for 3 to 6 months following drug-eluting stent implantation [8]. Despite the clear benefits of aspirin in the setting of PCI, a significant number of patients still suffer thrombotic complications. Among other explanations, recent investigations have demonstrated significant variability among the population with respect to antiplatelet response to aspirin therapy, or so-called "aspirin

resistance" [9]. Furthermore, the biochemical finding of aspirin resistance has been demonstrated, prospectively, to result in up to a threefold increase in the risk of major adverse outcome in patients who have established cardiovascular disease [10]. Although the complete details are not discussed in depth in this article, aspirin resistance exists in large part as a result of genetic heterogeneity and as a manifestation of the redundancy of the platelet thrombus pathway. It is this redundancy that is the target of the other therapies discussed in the following section.

Platelet ADP receptor antagonists

Thienopyridine antiplatelet agents including ticlopidine and clopidogrel are prodrugs that, when metabolized, achieve their antiplatelet effects by inhibiting the binding of ADP to its G protein–coupled P2Y12 purinergic receptor. When active, the P2Y12 receptor inhibits platelet disaggregation, an effect mediated by intracellular cyclic AMP [11]. Inhibition of this receptor, with the resultant impairment in platelet aggregation, provides the basis for the development and study of the current and future antiplatelet agents discussed in this section.

The use of thienopyridine platelet P2Y12 receptor antagonists paralleled the introduction of intracoronary stents to the interventional cardiology world. Routine stenting dramatically decreased the risk of abrupt or threatened vessel closure and restenosis [12]; however, it also led to concern over possible subacute thrombotic vessel occlusion due to the inherent thrombogenicity of the implanted intracoronary stent. These concerns resulted in several investigations regarding the optimal anticoagulation regimen after unplanned or elective stenting. In the STARS trial (see Appendix 1 for a glossary of clinical trial acronyms that appear in this article), 1653 patients were randomized to receive aspirin monotherapy, ticlopidine plus aspirin, or warfarin plus aspirin after intracoronary stenting. In this study, it was found that treatment with aspirin plus ticlopidine compared with aspirin alone or aspirin plus warfarin resulted in a lower rate of stent thrombosis [13]. Similar results were seen in the FANTASTIC study comparing ticlopidine plus aspirin versus warfarin plus aspirin after routine stenting. In addition to improved efficacy with the antiplatelet strategy, the additional finding of reduced bleeding was observed [14]. Multiple additional randomized trials in varying patient populations yielded consistent results, thus solidifying the role of dual antiplatelet therapy after PCI [15–17].

Despite the clear efficacy afforded by ticlopidine in addition to aspirin or in place of full anticoagulation after intracoronary stenting, ticlopidine is associated with a significant number of adverse effects that have ultimately limited its use. The most common serious side effect attributed to ticlopidine is severe drug-induced neutropenia. Occurring in 1% to 2% of patients, usually within the first 3 months of therapy, this potentially fatal side effect mandates immediate cessation of the drug [18]. A less common but potentially more serious adverse effect of ticlopidine is the development of thrombotic thrombocytopenic purpura–hemolytic uremic syndrome (TTP-HUS). Most often occurring 3 to 12 weeks after initiation of the drug, the frequency of this complication ranges from 1 in 1600 to 1 in 4800 patients treated. Like severe neutropenia, development of TTP-HUS necessitates immediate discontinuation of the drug and requires additional therapy with timely plasmapheresis [19,20]. As a result of these and other less specific adverse effects, ticlopidine has essentially been replaced by clopidogrel for the prevention of subacute stent thrombosis. The basis for this change (ie, the dramatically reduced incidence of side effects) was demonstrated in the CLASSICS trial that compared clopidogrel versus ticlopidine in addition to aspirin after PCI. Clopidogrel was associated with a 50% reduction in the incidence of the combined end point of major bleeding, thrombocytopenia, neutropenia, or discontinuation for noncardiac adverse events (4.6% versus 9.1%) [21].

In addition to a more favorable safety profile, clopidogrel may be more efficacious than ticlopidine. A large meta-analysis of trials and registries comparing clopidogrel and ticlopidine demonstrated reduced major adverse cardiac events with the use of clopidogrel (Fig. 2) [22]. One potential mechanism for differential efficacy is related to the onset of action of platelet inhibition, which is significantly slower with ticlopidine than with clopidogrel [23]. Platelet activation and distal embolization are major factors responsible for PCI-related ischemic complications, and because these events occur with initial vessel instrumentation, the issues of pretreatment and optimal loading dose of oral antiplatelet therapy have become particularly relevant.

The PCI subset of the CURE trial gave the initial indication that pretreatment with a 300-mg dose of clopidogrel was clinically useful. In the CURE trial, 12,562 patients who had acute coronary syndromes (ACS) were given aspirin plus loading and maintenance-therapy clopidogrel or placebo [24]. In the 2658 patients undergoing PCI who received the loading dose a median of 10 days before the procedure, the primary end point of cardiovascular death, MI, or urgent revascularization was significantly reduced in the clopidogrel pretreatment group (4.5% versus 6.4%), with no differences in major bleeding [25]. In the CREDO trial, 2100 patients were randomized to a loading dose of 300 mg of clopidogrel or placebo 3 to 24 hours before elective PCI. All subjects received 28 days of clopidogrel followed by 11 months of therapy dictated by the original randomization, with 40% receiving glycoprotein IIb/IIIa inhibition. In the pretreatment group, particularly in those who received clopidogrel more than 6 hours before PCI, there was a nearly significant reduction in 28-day death, MI, or urgent revascularization. At 1 year, there was a significant reduction in the combined end

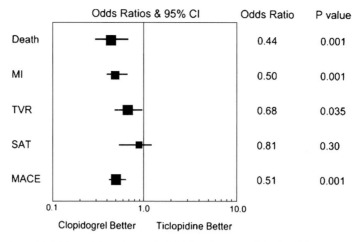

Fig. 2. Odds ratio plots with 95% confidence intervals (CIs) for the rates of death, MI, target vessel revascularization (TVR), subacute stent thrombosis (SAT), and major adverse cardiac events (MACE) using clopidogrel compared with ticlopidine after intracoronary stenting. (*From* Bhatt DL, Bertrand ME, Berger PB, et al. Meta-analysis of randomized and registry comparisons of ticlopidine with clopidogrel after stenting. J Am Coll Cardiol 2002;39(1):9–14; with permission.)

point of death, MI, or stroke in the loading and long-term clopidogrel treatment group (8.5% versus 11.5%), without a significant increase in major bleeding (Table 1). Subgroup analyses demonstrated that longer intervals between the 300-mg loading dose of clopidogrel and PCI may reduce events [26].

Universal pretreatment of patients with clopidogrel, however, has met with two major practical limitations. Specifically, in the CURE trial, the patients randomized to clopidogrel who underwent coronary bypass grafting within 5 days of receiving the drug had a 53% increased risk for

major bleeding compared with similar patients receiving placebo, presumably due to prolonged platelet inhibition [24]. This finding has led to reluctance to pretreat patients undergoing coronary angiography for fear of delaying revascularization in patients whose anatomy is more suitable for coronary artery bypass grafting. These concerns, however, may become less relevant because decreasing numbers of patients are being referred for surgical revascularization in the era of drug-eluting stents. The second issue limiting clopidogrel pretreatment relates to catheterization laboratory infrastructure and the feasibility of dosing

Table 1
One-year clinical outcomes for clopidogrel versus placebo from The Clopidogrel for The Reduction of Events During Observation trial

End point	Number of patients (%)		RRR (95% CI)
	Clopidogrel (n = 1053)	Placebo (n = 1063)	
Death, MI, stroke	89 (8.5)	122 (11.5)	26.9 (3.9–44.4)
Death, MI	84 (7.9)	111 (10.4)	24.0 (−0.9–42.7)
Death	18 (1.7)	24 (2.3)	24.6 (−38.9–59.1)
MI	70 (6.7)	89 (8.4)	20.8 (−8.4–42.1)
Stroke	9 (0.9)	10 (0.9)	10.0 (−21.3–24.0)
Revascularization			
Any TVR	138 (13.1)	144 (13.6)	4.0 (−21.3–24.0)
Urgent TVR	21 (2.0)	23 (2.2)	8.1 (−66.1–49.1)
Any revascularization	224 (21.3)	223 (21.0)	−1.1 (−21.7–16.0)

Abbreviations: CI, confidence interval; RRR, relative risk reduction; TVR, target vessel revascularization.
From Steinhubl SR, Tan WA, Foody JM, et al. Early and sustained dual oral antiplatelet therapy following percutaneous coronary intervention: a randomized controlled trial. JAMA 2002;288(19):2411–20; with permission.

patients several hours to days before their procedure. This issue is more directly addressed by numerous studies evaluating the pharmacodynamics of different loading doses of clopidogrel in human subjects. Specifically, it is clear that a higher loading dose of clopidogrel leads to more rapid and long-lasting inhibition of ADP-induced ex vivo platelet aggregation [27]. Further insight was gained from the ISAR-REACT trial in which low-risk elective PCI patients received a 600-mg loading dose of clopidogrel before PCI and were randomized to PCI with or without abciximab, with no significant difference in ischemic outcomes. In a prespecified subanalysis of the timing of pretreatment, there was no difference in the combined ischemic end point of death, MI, or urgent revascularization for abciximab versus placebo among patients receiving clopidogrel 2 to 3 hours, 3 to 6 hours, 6 to 12 hours, or more than 12 hours before PCI (Fig. 3) [28]. More recently, 300-mg versus 600-mg loading doses of clopidogrel were directly compared prospectively in the ARMYDA-2 trial. Patients who had stable or unstable angina scheduled for PCI were randomized to one of these two loading doses 4 to 8 hours before their procedure. The primary end point of death, MI, or urgent revascularization occurred significantly less often in the group receiving a 600-mg loading dose (4% versus 12%), although this difference was solely accounted for by a reduction in periprocedural MI [29]. The concept of a higher loading dose was advanced further by the recently reported ALBION trial

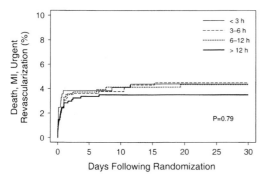

Fig. 3. Kaplan-Meier event curves for 30-day occurrence of death, MI, or urgent revascularization relative to clopidogrel loading-dose interval from the ISAR-RE-ACT study. (*From* Kandzari DE, Berger PB, Kastrati A, et al. Influence of treatment duration with a 600-mg dose of clopidogrel before percutaneous coronary revascularization. J Am Coll Cardiol 2004;44(11):2133–6; with permission.)

evaluating 103 patients who had ACS and received a 300-mg, 600-mg, or 900-mg loading dose of clopidogrel on presentation. Compared with the 300-mg loading dose, the 600-mg dose of clopidogrel demonstrated a more rapid onset of action and higher level of inhibition while maintaining a similar safety profile; 900 mg appeared to provide slightly higher antiplatelet inhibition than the 600 mg loading dose [30]. The ISAR-CHOICE study demonstrated additional platelet inhibition with a 600-mg loading dose versus a 300-mg loading dose, although 900 mg did not provide any further antiplatelet effect compared with the 600-mg loading dose in this study [31]. Further investigation of higher loading doses in the setting of PCI is ongoing.

Despite the almost universal use of dual antiplatelet agents in PCI, periprocedural ischemic complications still occur, and a small percentage (0.4%–1.1%) of patients suffer subacute stent thrombosis [32]. As is the case with aspirin, variability in response to clopidogrel is an increasingly recognized entity that may account for some of these events. Laboratory measurements demonstrate that up to 30% of patients may have an inadequate antiplatelet response to standard dosing of clopidogrel, a finding that correlates with cytochrome P450 3A4 metabolic activity, although this has not been correlated with clinical events per se [33]. As such, the search for more potent antiplatelet agents continues. One such agent is prasugrel, a novel oral thienopyridine that has more predictable and potent antiplatelet effects [34]. The JUMBO–TIMI 26 trial, a phase II dose-finding study of prasugrel versus clopidogrel in patients undergoing elective or urgent PCI, suggested an equivalent bleeding risk to clopidogrel, with a trend toward more efficacy at 30 days in the prasugrel-treated patients [35]. TRITON–TIMI 38, a large-scale randomized trial for efficacy of prasugrel versus clopidogrel in patients who have ACS undergoing PCI, is ongoing. Because thienopyridines are prodrugs that require metabolism to produce active metabolites, there is an inherent delay in their effect [11]. As such, development and investigation of nonthienopyridine direct P2Y12 receptor antagonists are also underway. AZD6140, a novel oral direct P2Y12 receptor antagonist, appears to be a more potent, consistent, and immediate platelet antagonist [36]. The DISPERSE-2 phase II trial evaluated this agent in patients who had ACS and found a similar rate of bleeding and similar ischemic events to clopidogrel, although there was a higher rate of dyspnea with AZD6140 [37]. Cangrelor, an analog of the endogenous direct platelet ADP receptor inhibitor ATP, is an intravenous drug demonstrating more immediate antiplatelet effects. Initial studies suggest consistent, rapid, and potent platelet inhibition and an acceptable safety profile [36]. Larger clinical trials of this intravenous agent are planned.

Although CREDO and PCI-CURE support the use of clopidogrel in addition to aspirin for a year after PCI, longer-term therapy may yield even greater benefit. This issue is being addressed as part of the ongoing CHARISMA trial [38]. The issue of prolonged dual antiplatelet therapy may be particularly relevant with drug-eluting stents, which seem to have the potential for delayed stent thrombosis compared with bare metal stents when antiplatelet therapy is interrupted (such as for surgery) or discontinued.

Platelet glycoprotein IIb/IIIa receptor antagonists

Although platelets can be activated by a number of different pharmacologic and mechanical stimuli, their ability to aggregate and adhere to disrupted endothelium is largely mediated by the surface glycoprotein IIb/IIIa receptor, a member of the integrin family of membrane receptors [39]. With activation, the surface expression and conformation of the glycoprotein IIb/IIIa receptor changes, rendering it competent to bind a number of different ligands. Fibrinogen, by far the dominant ligand, is bound by the activated glycoprotein IIb/IIIa receptor at opposite ends, allowing a cross-link to form between two adjacent platelets and the endothelium [40]. This common pathway for platelet aggregation and adherence has served as a potentially high-yielding target in the development of antiplatelet agents for PCI.

Currently, there are three intravenous glycoprotein IIb/IIIa inhibitors available clinically: abciximab, tirofiban, and eptifibatide. Features of the different intravenous glycoprotein IIb/IIIa receptor antagonists are summarized in Table 2. All of these agents have been studied extensively in large clinical trials, the results of which are discussed in the following sections.

Abciximab

Originally produced in 1985 and subsequently approved by the Food and Drug Administration (FDA) in 1994, abciximab is the Fab antibody fragment of a chimeric human-murine monoclonal antibody specific for the glycoprotein IIb/IIIa receptor. Joined with the constant regions of human immunoglobulin, this chimer allows for preserved specificity with minimal antigenicity [41]. Initial animal and human pilot studies verified the potent antiplatelet effect of abciximab with up to 93% platelet inhibition at 2 hours in patients receiving the highest dose [42,43]. Clinical efficacy was demonstrated on completion of the EPIC trial, the original large experience with abciximab in the catheterization laboratory. In this study, 2099 high-risk patients undergoing PTCA or atherectomy were randomized to abciximab or placebo in addition to receiving aspirin and heparin. Patients randomized to a bolus of abciximab followed by a 12-hour infusion had a 35% reduction in the primary composite end point of death, MI, or urgent intervention at 30 days. These benefits were maintained at 6 months and at 3 years and were greatest in magnitude in those who had evolving MI [44,45]. The EPILOG trial, another large trial solidifying the efficacy of abciximab in PCI, randomized patients undergoing elective or urgent PCI to abciximab plus standard- or low-dose

Table 2
Dosing and pharmacokinetic comparison of clinically available intravenous glycoprotein IIb-IIIa inhibitors

Feature	Abciximab	Eptifibatide	Tirofiban
Mechanism	Chimeric antibody	Cyclic heptapeptide inhibitor	Nonpeptide inhibitor
Dose: loading	0.25 mg/kg × 1	180 μ/kg × 2 (10-min interval)	0.4 μ/kg/min × 30 min[a]
Dose: infusion	0.125 μ/kg/min × 12 h	2 μ/kg/min × 18–24 h	0.1 μ/kg/min × 18–24 h[a]
Plasma half-life	30 min	2.5 h	2 h
Dose reduction in CRI	None	Load: None Infusion: 50% (CrCl < 50 mL/min)	Load: 50% Infusion: 50% (CrCl < 30 mL/min)
Reversible with platelet infusion	Yes	No	No
Removed by hemodialysis	No	Yes	Yes

Abbreviations: CrCl, creatinine clearance; CRI, chronic renal insufficiency.
[a] FDA, approved dose for ACS.

adjunctive heparin or to placebo plus standard-dose heparin. The trial was halted prematurely after enrolling 2792 patients because the composite end point was significantly reduced in both abciximab groups compared with placebo. The treatment effect was seen in high- and low-risk individuals and was maintained at 6 months and at 1 year [46,47]. Validation for abciximab in the setting of intracoronary stenting came from the EPISTENT trial, a 2399-patient randomized study of stenting alone, abciximab plus stenting, or abciximab plus PTCA. Abciximab-treated patients demonstrated a significantly lower incidence of death, MI, or urgent revascularization at 30 days and at 6 months [48,49]. In addition, the beneficial effects of stenting plus abciximab on death and large MI were sustained at 1 year [50]. Pooled analysis of these three large randomized trials confirmed that the benefits of abciximab on 30-day death or MI are irrespective of sex or the PCI device used [51]. More important, the significant mortality benefit observed at short-term follow-up is durable, with an absolute risk reduction for death of 1.4% at 3 years (Fig. 4) [52].

The concept that selective patient populations derive a greater clinical benefit from the use of abciximab arose early in the evaluation of the drug. In the CAPTURE trial, for instance, 1265 patients who had medically refractory non–ST elevation ACS were randomized to receive abciximab versus placebo 18 to 24 hours before PTCA.

The benefit observed in this trial was predominantly limited to patients who had complex lesions on angiography or elevated serum troponin levels [53]. A similar finding was observed on analysis of the subset of patients in the EPISTENT trial who had complex atherosclerotic lesions [54]. In addition to patients who have complex lesions, post hoc analyses suggested that abciximab may be of particular benefit in those who have diabetes. In a pooled analysis of the 1462 patients who had diabetes enrolled in the EPIC, EPILOG, and EPISTENT trials, abciximab reduced their 1-year mortality to that observed in patients who did not have diabetes and were treated with placebo (Fig. 5) [55]. To date, however, the ISAR–SWEET trial has been the only large prospective trial to evaluate abciximab specifically in patients who have diabetes. In this trial, 701 patients receiving 600 mg of clopidogrel at least 2 hours before planned PCI were randomly assigned to abciximab or placebo with heparin. Although there was reduced angiographic restenosis and target vessel revascularization in the abciximab-treated group, there was no difference in the incidence of death or MI at 1 year in this study [56]. A potential explanation for the reduced restenosis rates observed in this and a number of the other abciximab trials relates to the effects that the drug may have on the vitronectin receptor and subsequent neointimal proliferation [57]. A prospective trial of 225 patients, however, found no difference between abciximab and placebo on neointimal proliferation as measured by

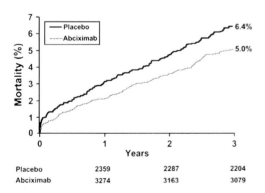

Fig. 4. Cumulative mortality at 3-year follow-up of abciximab-versus placebo-treated patients in the combined EPIC, EPILOG, and EPISTENT trials: intention-to-treat analysis. The differences were statistically significant (hazard ratio = 0.78; 95% confidence interval: 0.63–0.98; $P = 0.03$). (*From* Topol EJ, Lincoff AM, Kereiakes DJ, et al. Multi-year follow-up of abciximab therapy in three randomized, placebo-controlled trials of percutaneous coronary revascularization. Am J Med 2002;113(1):1–6; with permission.)

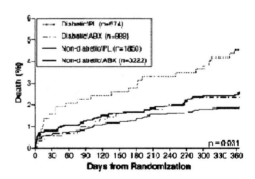

Fig. 5. Kaplan-Meier curves, pooled from the EPIC, EPILOG, and EPISTENT trials, for 1-year mortality in diabetics and nondiabetics randomized to placebo (PL) or abciximab (ABX). (*From* Bhatt DL, Marso SP, Loncoff AM, et al. Abciximab reduces mortality in diabetics following percutaneous coronary intervention. J Am Coll Cardiol 2000;35(4):922–8; with permission.)

intravascular ultrasound or quantitative angiography [58].

One group of patients who may not derive a detectable benefit from the routine use of abciximab includes those who are adequately pretreated with clopidogrel and who are at particularly low risk. The ISAR–REACT trial evaluated such patients. In this trial, pretreatment with 600 mg of clopidogrel for a median of 7.4 hours seemed to negate any beneficial effects of abciximab on death, MI, or urgent revascularization at 30 days [28]. Evaluation of high-dose pretreatment in higher-risk patients and the implications that this strategy may have on the utility of abciximab and other glycoprotein IIb/IIIa inhibitors is ongoing in the ISAR–REACT-2 study.

Despite the decreasing number of patients suffering ST-segment elevation MI (STEMI) annually, it remains an important subset presenting to the catheterization laboratory. The use of abciximab as adjunctive pharmacotherapy in patients who have STEMI undergoing primary angioplasty has also been extensively studied; most of these studies suggest benefit of abciximab in this setting. In the ADMIRAL trial, 300 patients were randomized to placebo or abciximab before PTCA or stenting. The primary composite end point of death, MI, or revascularization was significantly lower at 30 days and at 6 months in the abciximab group. In addition, TIMI-3 flow rates at initial catheterization and 6-month left ventricular ejection fraction were higher in the abciximab group. These benefits were enhanced in the subset of patients who received abciximab earlier (ie, in the ambulance or emergency room), a finding subsequently supported by a meta-analysis of six large trials of glycoprotein IIb/IIIa inhibition in primary PCI [59,60]. Evaluation at 3-year follow up confirmed the durability of benefit of abciximab treatment by demonstrating a 3.1% absolute risk reduction in all-cause mortality (9.1% versus 12.2%) [61]. Similar beneficial findings were observed in the ISAR-2, RAPPORT, and ACE trials [62–65]. The largest trial of abciximab in STEMI patients, the CADILLAC trial, resulted in much less benefit with abciximab. In this trial, 2082 patients were randomized in a two-by-two factorial design to placebo or abciximab and PTCA or stenting. The 6-month composite end point of death, MI, or ischemia-driven revascularization was lower with stenting compared with PTCA, irrespective of abciximab use. Angiographic restenosis was also lower with stenting, again with or without abciximab [66]. As a result of the somewhat conflicting results seen in the CADILLAC trial, which may have been related to study design and the exclusion of sicker patients, a meta-analysis was performed of trials evaluating abciximab in patients who had STEMI treated with fibrinolysis and primary PCI. This analysis demonstrated significant reductions in mortality at 30 days (2.4% versus 3.4%) and between 6 and 12 months (4.4% versus 6.2%), without an increase in significant bleeding, a benefit seen only in patients undergoing primary PCI but not in those receiving fibrinolysis (Fig. 6) [67]. These data provide strong support for abciximab before primary angioplasty for STEMI.

Although the efficacy of abciximab is clear, several features may limit its use. In particular, acute profound thrombocytopenia resulting from antibody formation, prolonged antiplatelet effect given the relatively long half-life, and cost have caused concern. As such, two other glycoprotein IIb/IIIa inhibitors, eptifibatide and tirofiban, have been studied in the setting of PCI.

Eptifibatide

Eptifibatide, first approved by the FDA in 1998, is a nonimmunogenic cyclic heptapeptide derived from the structure of barbourin, a platelet glycoprotein IIb/IIIa inhibitor found in the venom of the southeastern pigmy rattlesnake. Initial pilot studies of the medication suggested that a bolus dose between 135 to 180 µg/kg was sufficient to block 80% of ADP-mediated platelet aggregation within 15 minutes of administration, with various continuous infusions sustaining the effect [68,69]. The PURSUIT trial evaluated the 180-µg/kg bolus dose of eptifibatide along with a high- or low-infusion dose versus placebo in patients who had ACS. In this high-risk patient population, 46% of whom had non-STEMI, eptifibatide therapy was associated with a lower incidence of death or nonfatal MI at 30 days (14.2% versus 15.7%) [70]. Although the benefit was seen across all groups, it was observed that those undergoing early PCI derived a larger benefit [71]. Eptifibatide therapy in patients specifically undergoing PCI was addressed in the IMPACT-II trial. In this study, 4010 patients undergoing planned, urgent, or emergent PCI were randomized to placebo or a bolus of eptifibatide and one of two infusion doses before PCI. At 30 days, the incidence of the composite end point of death, MI, unplanned revascularization, or

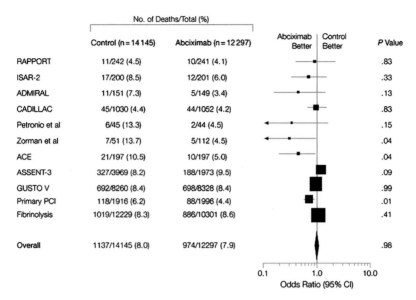

No. of Deaths/Total (%)

	Control (n = 14 145)	Abciximab (n = 12 297)	Abciximab Better / Control Better	P Value
RAPPORT	11/242 (4.5)	10/241 (4.1)		.83
ISAR-2	17/200 (8.5)	12/201 (6.0)		.33
ADMIRAL	11/151 (7.3)	5/149 (3.4)		.13
CADILLAC	45/1030 (4.4)	44/1052 (4.2)		.83
Petronio et al	6/45 (13.3)	2/44 (4.5)		.15
Zorman et al	7/51 (13.7)	5/112 (4.5)		.04
ACE	21/197 (10.5)	10/197 (5.0)		.04
ASSENT-3	327/3969 (8.2)	188/1973 (9.5)		.09
GUSTO V	692/8260 (8.4)	698/8328 (8.4)		.99
Primary PCI	118/1916 (6.2)	88/1996 (4.4)		.01
Fibrinolysis	1019/12229 (8.3)	886/10301 (8.6)		.41
Overall	1137/14145 (8.0)	974/12297 (7.9)		.98

0.1   1.0   10.0
Odds Ratio (95% CI)

Fig. 6. Incidence of and odds ratio plots with 95% confidence intervals (CIs) for 6- to 12-month mortality with abciximab compared with placebo from trials of primary angioplasty and fibrinolysis in the treatment of STEMI. The size of the data markers (*squares*) is approximately proportional to the sample size of each treatment group. (*From* De Luca G, Suryapranata H, Stone GW, et al. Abciximab as adjunctive therapy to reperfusion in acute ST-segment elevation myocardial infarction: a meta-analysis of randomized trials. JAMA 2005;293(14):1759–65; with permission.)

stent placement for abrupt vessel closure was significantly decreased in the eptifibatide plus lower-dose-infusion group. The treatment benefit observed, however, was not maintained at 6 months [72]. The proposed explanation for the lack of durable efficacy in the IMPACT-II trial was the fact that the bolus and infusion doses studied were lower than those used in the PURSUIT trial. Indeed, only 50% of maximal platelet inhibition was achieved in the IMPACT-II trial [73]. Subsequent study established the biochemical efficacy of a novel, double-bolus strategy of eptifibatide before PCI [74]. This dosing strategy provided the basis for the dosing in the ESPRIT trial that evaluated 2064 patients scheduled for elective PCI and ultimately confirmed the efficacy of eptifibatide before PCI. In the ESPRIT trial, patients were randomized to double-bolus eptifibatide plus continuous infusion or to placebo. The trial was terminated prematurely because there was a large decrease in the primary end point of death, MI, urgent revascularization, or thrombotic bailout use of glycoprotein IIb/IIIa inhibitor therapy within 48 hours in the eptifibatide group compared with placebo. The results were durable to 1 year and were consistent among all subgroups analyzed (Fig. 7) [75–77]. The safety of eptifibatide is well established. Although there was an increased need for transfusion in eptifibatide-treated patients in the PURSUIT trial, pooled analysis has not demonstrated an increased risk of thrombocytopenia or of hemorrhagic stroke, the most devastating potential complication of periprocedural antithrombotic therapy [78]. Given the findings of the ESPRIT trial and the cumulative safety data, double-bolus plus higher-dose continuous infusion of eptifibatide has become the standard dose for patients receiving this glycoprotein IIb/IIIa inhibitor as adjunctive pharmacotherapy in the setting of coronary stent implantation.

Tirofiban

The third intravenous glycoprotein IIb/IIIa inhibitor used in clinical practice is tirofiban, which also was approved by the FDA in 1998. The pharmacokinetic features of this nonpeptide competitive inhibitor of the glycoprotein IIb/IIIa inhibitor are given in Table 2. Phase I study of the drug identified the optimal bolus and infusion dose to achieve significant and sustained platelet inhibition as measured by an ex vivo platelet aggregation assay [79]. It also provided the basis for the dosing of tirofiban in the RESTORE trial, the first large randomized trial of the drug in PCI.

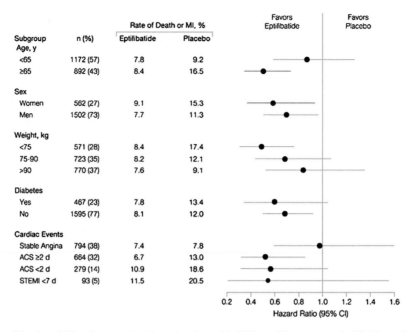

Subgroup	n (%)	Rate of Death or MI, %	
Age, y		Eptifibatide	Placebo
<65	1172 (57)	7.8	9.2
≥65	892 (43)	8.4	16.5
Sex			
Women	562 (27)	9.1	15.3
Men	1502 (73)	7.7	11.3
Weight, kg			
<75	571 (28)	8.4	17.4
75-90	723 (35)	8.2	12.1
>90	770 (37)	7.6	9.1
Diabetes			
Yes	467 (23)	7.8	13.4
No	1595 (77)	8.1	12.0
Cardiac Events			
Stable Angina	794 (38)	7.4	7.8
ACS ≥2 d	664 (32)	6.7	13.0
ACS <2 d	279 (14)	10.9	18.6
STEMI <7 d	93 (5)	11.5	20.5

Fig. 7. Rates of death or MI at 1 year and odds ratio plots with 95% confidence intervals (CIs) in various subgroups from the ESPRIT trial. (*From* O'Shea JC, Butler CE, Cantor WJ, et al. Long-term efficacy of platelet glycoprotein IIb/ IIIa integrin blockade with eptifibatide in coronary stent intervention. JAMA 2002;287(5):618–21; with permission.)

Randomizing 2139 patients who had ACS and were undergoing PCI within 72 hours, the RE-STORE trial evaluated tirofiban versus placebo. The composite end point of death, MI, failed angioplasty requiring bypass surgery, urgent revascularization, or implantation of an intracoronary stent because of actual or threatened abrupt closure was lower in the tirofiban group compared with placebo at 30-day (10.3% versus 12.2%) and at 6-month follow-up (24.1% versus 27.1%), although the differences were not statistically significant [80,81]. In the PRISM-PLUS trial, 1915 patients who had ACS were randomized to receive heparin only, tirofiban only, or tirofiban plus heparin. Patients underwent angioplasty after 48 hours of drug treatment at the discretion of the treating physician. Randomization to the tirofiban-only arm was discontinued early because this group demonstrated increased mortality at 7 days. The group treated with tirofiban and heparin, however, had a significant reduction in the incidence of death, MI, or refractory ischemia at 7 days (12.9% versus 17.9%), an effect that was maintained at 30 days (18.5% versus 22.3%) and at 6 months (27.7% versus 32.1%). The benefits of tirofiban with heparin were seen in patients who were treated medically and in those who underwent angioplasty [82]. In addition, from PRISM-PLUS, five independent clinical risk factors that predicted benefit from tirofiban therapy were identified. Consistent with other trials of glycoprotein IIb/IIIa inihibitors that demonstrated increasing benefit in sicker patients, those who had 0 or 1 risk factors had no detectable advantage from tirofiban therapy, whereas those who had more risk factors demonstrated a clear and increasing benefit (Fig. 8) [83]. Despite the validation of tirofiban in patients who have ACS, the lack of a significant durable benefit in the RESTORE trial has limited its use in coronary patients undergoing planned PCI. As with eptifibatide, issues of dosing and the limitations of ex vivo platelet aggregation studies as an accurate surrogate of in vivo inhibition served as the potential explanation for the relatively weaker efficacy of tirofiban in the catheterization laboratory. The ADVANCE trial attempted to resolve this issue. This smaller study randomized 202 patients to high-dose bolus tirofiban and infusion versus placebo on a baseline of heparin and aspirin. At 6 months, the primary composite end point of death, MI, or target vessel revascularization was significantly lower in the high-dose tirofiban group (20% versus 35%). Subgroup analysis suggested that the benefits of tirofiban in this study were limited to those who had ACS and those

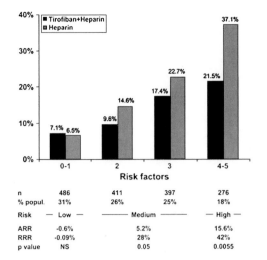

n	486	411	397	276
% popul.	31%	26%	25%	18%
Risk	— Low —	Medium	— High —
ARR	-0.6%	5.2%	15.6%
RRR	-0.09%	28%	42%
p value	NS	0.05	0.0055

Fig. 8. Composite event rate of death, MI, or refractory ischemia at 7 days for patients from the PRISM-PLUS trial stratified by risk factor score and treatment group. One point assigned to risk factor score for each of the following: age greater than 65 years, prior bypass surgery, antecedent aspirin use, antecedent β-blocker use, and ST depressions on the presenting electrocardiogram. ARR, absolute risk reduction; NS, not significant; % popul., percentage of patients in each risk score group; RRR, relative risk reduction. (*From* Sabatine MS, Januzzi JL, Snapinn S, et al. A risk score system for predicting adverse outcomes and magnitude of benefit with glycoprotein IIb/IIIa inhibitor therapy in patients with unstable angina pectoris. Am J Cardiol 2001;88(5):488–92; with permission.)

who had diabetes [84]. At present, the use of tirofiban in most catheterization laboratories remains limited to those patients who have ACS and are already receiving the drug.

The use of glycoprotein IIb/IIIa inhibitors in specific circumstances also merits close consideration. For instance, in saphenous vein graft intervention, the role of these agents is much less well established. A pooled analysis of five large randomized trials including 627 patients undergoing saphenous vein graft intervention failed to demonstrate any benefit of glycoprotein IIb/IIIa inhibition [85]. Although there may be a role for these agents in saphenous vein graft interventions using emboli protection devices, this concept requires further study before it can be clearly recommended. Patients who have impaired renal function also represent a population in whom the utility of glycoprotein IIb/IIIa inhibition is less firmly grounded. The issue is relevant because this condition is increasingly prevalent and these

patients are generally at higher risk. Dose reduction of renally cleared glycoprotein IIb/IIIa inhibitors has been established, as has efficacy, albeit by way of post hoc analysis. Prospective study in this group is still necessary. Lastly, because most trials of glycoprotein IIb/IIIa inhibitors occurred during a time of balloon angioplasty and bare metal stenting, their utility in the current era of drug-eluting stenting must be inferred. Biologically, there is unlikely to be a difference in the setting of bare metal versus drug-eluting stenting because delivery systems and technique are similar; however, because repeat prospective trials are not forthcoming, analysis of registry data is important to evaluate this question.

Overall, the general use of glycoprotein IIb/IIIa inhibition with PCI is well supported by the literature. A meta-analysis of 19 large randomized trials of glycoprotein IIb/IIIa inhibitors in a variety of different patient populations confirmed a significant reduction in mortality at 30 days (relative risk reduction = 0.69) and at 6 months (relative risk reduction = 0.79) compared with placebo. The reduction in the risk of mortality is only partially explained by reduction in MI [86]. The extent of benefit is clearly related to patient features, with high-risk patients generally deriving a greater degree of benefit. Patients who have diabetes and ACS especially seem to benefit from glycoprotein IIb/IIIa inhibitor use, presumably because they are generally at an increased state of platelet activation [87,88]. On the contrary, low-risk patients undergoing elective stenting, particularly those who have been adequately pretreated with clopidogrel with respect to timing and dose, may not benefit from adjunctive glycoprotein IIb/IIIa inhibition. As far as comparative efficacy is concerned, a separate meta-analysis evaluated the efficacy and safety of the three agents. Obviously limited by the included study designs, this study suggested superiority of abciximab compared with eptifibatide and tirofiban with respect to MI and target vessel revascularization at the cost of increased bleeding [89]. To date, however, only 1 prospective randomized trial exists comparing two agents. In the TARGET trial, 4809 patients were randomized to receive abciximab or tirofiban before nonemergent stent implantation. Designed to test for noninferiority of tirofiban, this study found instead that abciximab was significantly superior in terms of the primary end point of death, MI, or urgent revascularization at 30 days (6% versus 7.6%) [90]. Ultimately, the decision of which agent to use as adjunctive pharmacotherapy in PCI rests on the operator. The EPISTENT and ESPRIT trials support the use of abciximab and eptifibatide, respectively, in the setting of elective stenting. The use of tirofiban in this setting is less well established and may be a result of suboptimal dosing.

Another intravenous agent, lamifaban, with potentially advantageous pharmacokinetics was developed as a possible replacement to the current glycoprotein IIb/IIIa agents being used. The safety and efficacy of this nonpeptide inhibitor was evaluated in the Canadian Lamifaban Study and in PARAGON A and B, clinical trials that enrolled patients who had ACS. Although these studies suggested potential benefit of this medication, there is no plan to continue development of this agent [91–93]. In addition, no large dedicated study of this agent in patients undergoing planned PCI has been performed. Oral glycoprotein IIb/IIIa inhibitors, although extensively studied, are discussed only briefly because they currently have no clinical utility. Initially holding promise, multiple trials of these oral agents yielded disappointing results. A meta-analysis of four large studies of patients treated with oral glycoprotein IIb/IIIa inhibitors for 3 to 6 months, including more than 33,000 patients, not only demonstrated a clear lack of efficacy but also suggested increased mortality in addition to increased rates of major bleeding with their use (Fig. 9) [94]. The mechanism of the clinical failure of these agents is still unclear.

Anticoagulants

It has long been known that antiplatelets alone cannot substantially reduce platelet activation in an environment of high thrombin activity. Because vessel injury during PCI induces a substantial amount of thrombin generation through TF activation of the coagulation cascade, the concomitant use of antithrombotic therapy during this procedure has been intuitive.

Unfractionated and low molecular weight heparin

Unfractionated heparin (UFH) has been used in the setting of PCI for over 20 years to prevent periprocedural ischemic complications. By binding circulating antithrombin, UFH induces a conformation change that results in accelerated inactivation of several coagulation factors, particularly factor Xa. Inhibition of factor IIa, thrombin, occurs when larger molecular weight fractions of

heparin form a tertiary complex by binding to thrombin and to antithrombin. Given the variable dose-response relationship of heparin (a result of drug composition inconsistencies and patient variations of antithrombin activity), monitoring of drug effect is essential. Because the activated partial thromboplastin time is greatly prolonged with high-dose heparin use, the activated clotting time (ACT) has become the standard by which the UFH effect is measured in the catheterization laboratory [95]. Despite its widespread use, a dramatic absence of large-scale, well-conducted prospective studies evaluating UFH in PCI exists. In response to this lack of evidence, a pooled analysis of six large randomized trials of novel anticoagulants, in which UFH was used in the control arm, was conducted to characterize the efficacy of heparin in PCI and to describe the optimal ACT for its use. In this analysis, an ACT of 350 to 375 seconds was associated with the lowest ischemic event rate at 7 days after PCI. Because an ACT between 325 and 350 seconds was associated with lower rates of bleeding, it is more widely accepted as the target ACT during coronary interventions in which UFH is the primary anticoagulant (Fig. 10) [96]. When UFH is used adjunctively with glycoprotein IIb/IIIa inhibitors, the target ACT is significantly lower. A large meta-analysis including 8369 patients who had available ACT data (89% of whom received concominant glycoprotein IIb/IIIa inhibition) suggested that the incidence of death, MI, or target vessel revascularization was equivalent in patients whose ACTs were less than 256, 257 to 296, 297 to 347, or greater than 348 seconds. The risk of bleeding, however, was found to increase with increasing ACT [97]. From these data, it is generally accepted that the goal ACT to achieve maximal safety and efficacy, when concominant glycoprotein IIb/IIIa inhibitors are used, is between 200 and 250 seconds. With respect to duration of therapy, it was common in the initial era of PTCA to continue UFH for up to 24 hours after the procedure [98]. At the cost of increased bleeding and prolonged hospitalization, it was originally believed that prolonged therapy might reduce postprocedural ischemic events. With the advent of stents and more effective long-term oral antiplatelet agents, however, subacute ischemic events have substantially decreased, and UFH therapy after coronary intervention is no longer recommended [99].

Despite continuing to be the predominant antithrombotic used during PCI, UFH has several major limitations that have led to the search for

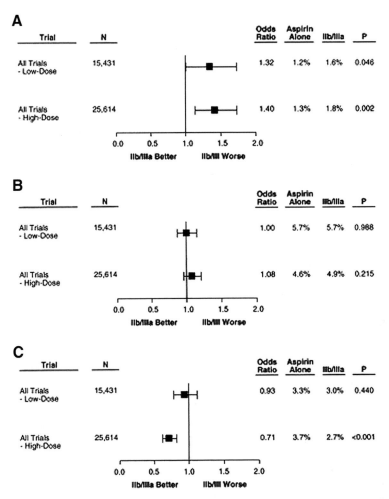

Fig. 9. Odds ratios and 95% confidence intervals for risk of death (*A*), MI (*B*), and urgent revascularization (*C*) beyond 30 days with respect to low-dose oral glycoprotein IIb/IIIa inhibitor versus aspirin alone and high-dose oral glycoprotein IIb/IIIa inhibitor versus aspirin alone. N indicates sample size. (*From* Chew DP, Bhatt DL, Sapp S, et al. Increased mortality with oral platelet glycoprotein IIb/IIIa antagonists: a meta-analysis of phase III multicenter randomized trials. Circulation 2001;103(2):201–6; with permission.)

alternative agents. In particular, UFH has a narrow therapeutic index with a highly variable dose-response relationship. It is unable to inhibit thrombin bound to fibrin, thus allowing existing thrombus to grow. In addition, UFH may actually promote platelet aggregation, potentially explaining the observed rebound hypercoaguability seen when it is discontinued. Lastly, it has been increasingly recognized that some patients may suffer significant heparin-induced thrombocytopenia with re-exposure, a potentially fatal complication that can paradoxically be associated with systemic thrombosis. In response to these limitations, the development and study of low molecular weight heparins (LMWH), fragments of UFH

prepared by chemical or enzymatic depolymerization, has been extensive. By predominantly inhibiting factor Xa, as opposed to thrombin directly, LMWH inhibits upstream activation of the coagulation cascade, thus acting more efficiently and avoiding many of the limitations of UFH. LMWHs are more easily administered, have a more reliable anticoagulant effect, and are associated with fewer side effects than UFH [100,101]. As such, these agents, of which enoxaparin is the most common, have been evaluated in the setting of ACS and PCI.

In an early trial comparing intravenous LMWH to intravenous UFH in PCI, 60 patients received a 1-mg/kg dose of enoxaparin or UFH,

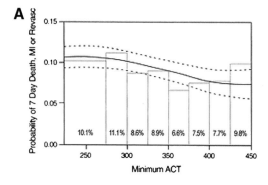

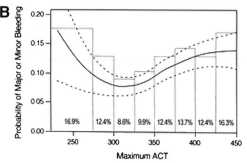

Fig. 10. (*A*) Relationship between minimum ACT at or around time of device activation and death, MI, or urgent revascularization (Revasc) at 7 days. (*B*) Relationship between maximum ACT and major or minor bleeding events at 7 days. Lowest smoothing estimate and 95% confidence intervals indicated by solid and dotted lines, respectively. Percentages represent actual event rates observed. (*From* Chew DP, Bhatt DL, Lincoff AM, et al. Defining the optimal activated clotting time during percutaneous coronary intervention: aggregate results from 6 randomized, controlled trials. Circulation 2001;103(7):961–6; with permission.)

with repeat boluses as needed, to maintain an ACT greater than 300 seconds. This small study demonstrated comparable levels of factor Xa inhibition and clinical outcomes, thus providing a basis for dosing of intravenous enoxaparin in the catheterization laboratory [102]. Although this and other small initial studies suggested benefit, clinical efficacy and safety of enoxaparin in the PCI was more firmly established by the NICE registry. In the NICE-1 study, 828 patients undergoing elective or urgent PCI receiving 1 mg/kg of intravenous enoxaparin at the time of the procedure were found (at 30 days) to be comparable to historical controls receiving UFH in terms of bleeding, death, MI, or urgent target vessel revascularization. Similarly, in the setting of abciximab therapy for elective or urgent PCI, the NICE-4 trial demonstrated that outcomes in patients

receiving a reduced dose of intravenous enoxaparin (0.75 mg/kg) were comparable to outcomes of historical controls from the EPILOG and EPISTENT trials who received UFH with abciximab [103,104]. The CRUISE trial provided more robust, prospective randomized data that suggested the efficacy and safety of enoxaparin with glycoprotein IIb/IIIa inhibition in elective PCI. In this trial, 261 patients receiving eptifibatide were randomized to receive 0.75 mg/kg of intravenous enoxaparin or UFH with their procedure. Clinical outcomes at 48 hours were similar in the two groups, with the enoxaparin group demonstrating a slight trend toward decreased bleeding (4.1% versus 10.5%) [105]. More recently, the STEEPLE study, which randomized 3528 patients undergoing elective PCI to UFH or one of two doses of enoxaparin, supported this trend of improved safety. Specifically, the enoxaparin group receiving a 0.75-mg/kg dose at the time of PCI had a lower major bleeding rate compared with the UFH group (1.2% versus 2.8%) [106].

The use of subcutaneous enoxaparin became an accepted strategy for the medical therapy for ACS after the completion of two large randomized trials in the late 1990s [107,108]. To address the issue of additional enoxaparin dosing at the time of PCI, the NICE-3 trial evaluated 628 patients being treated with subcutaneous enoxaparin and a glycoprotein IIb/IIIa inhibitor; 283 went on to PCI. Patients who received a subcutaneous enoxaparin dose between 8 and 12 hours before PCI were given an additional intravenous bolus of 0.3 mg/kg, whereas those who received a dose within 8 hours were given no additional anticoagulation. Again, compared with historical controls receiving heparin and a glycoprotein IIb/IIIa inhibitor, there was no significant difference in the incidence of death, MI, or bleeding related to non–coronary artery bypass grafting [109]. Evaluating this prospectively, the INTERACT study randomized patients who had ACS and who received eptifibatide and aspirin to subcutaneous enoxaparin or to UFH for 48 hours. In the two thirds of patients who ultimately proceeded to coronary angiography, nearly half underwent PCI. Patients in the enoxaparin group suffered significantly lower rates of bleeding and recurrent ischemic events at 48 and 96 hours. In addition, there was a lowering of the composite end point of death and reinfarction at 30 days in the group receiving enoxaparin (5.0% versus 9.0%) (Fig. 11) [110]. Although upstream use of LMWH in ACS is accepted, the strategy of

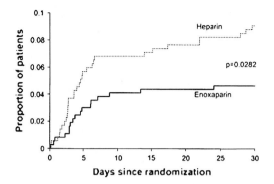

Fig. 11. Kaplan-Meier curves for the composite outcome of death or nonfatal myocardial reinfarction during the first 30 days after randomization in patients treated with UFH versus enoxaparin. (*From* Goodman SG, Fitchett D, Armstrong PW, et al. Randomized evaluation of the safety and efficacy of enoxaparin versus unfractionated heparin in high-risk patients with non-ST-segment elevation acute coronary syndromes receiving the glycoprotein IIb/IIIa inhibitor eptifibatide. Circulation 2003;107(2):238–44; with permission.)

continued LMWH therapy after PCI is much less well established. In a number of studies evaluating this question, in terms of reduced restenosis and subacute stent thrombosis, particularly in the setting of dual antiplatelet therapy, LMWH has not seemed to provide any additional benefit [111–115]. It is therefore not routinely recommended.

Despite a more predictable anticoagulant dose response, which may obviate the need for monitoring in most cases, a rapid point-of-care monitoring system would still likely improve the safety and efficacy of LMWH in the catheterization laboratory. Particularly in patients who have weight extremes or renal insufficiency, such a test might also guide timing of safe vascular sheath removal and administration of protamine for clinical bleeding (although protamine only reverses ~40% of enoxaparin activity). Indeed, the ELECT trial, a nonrandomized observational study of 445 patients, aimed to assess the predictive value of the ENOX test, a surrogate measure of anti-Xa activity. Patients in this trial who had an ENOX time within the proposed target range of 250 to 450 seconds had a 4% combined ischemic and bleeding event rate compared with 7.2% in patients outside of this range [116]. Despite FDA approval, however, this test of enoxaparin effect is unlikely to receive widespread clinical acceptance until it is validated in prospective trials.

The SYNERGY trial demonstrated the noninferiority of enoxaparin versus UFH in more than 10,000 patients who had ACS generally treated with an early invasive strategy. A significant proportion underwent PCI while on enoxaparin, and the rate of thrombotic complications was similar to that seen with UFH. A strategy of switching from enoxaparin to UFH or vice versa was associated with an increased hazard of bleeding [117].

Despite the limitation of readily quantifying effect, LMWH remains a reasonable choice for anticoagulation in patients undergoing PCI. It should be understood, however, that most clinical trials establishing the efficacy of this class of agents have used enoxaparin or dalteparin. Currently, there are seven clinically evaluated LWMHs, each with different ratios of factor Xa to IIa inhibition, and further investigation is necessary to justify their individual use.

Direct thrombin inhibitors

Direct thrombin inhibitors represent another major class of antithrombotics studied in the setting of PCI. These agents do not require binding to antithrombin to exert their anticoagulant effect because they directly inhibit the catalytic site on thrombin. Direct thrombin inhibitors inhibit soluble and clot-bound thrombin, a major potential advantage over heparin [118]. Other advantages over heparin include the fact that these agents do not activate platelets, do not bind plasma proteins, and are resistant to neutralization by platelet factors [119]. These features and the noncompetitive and reversible nature by which direct thrombin inhibitors binds thrombin allow for predictable, intense anticoagulation for a controlled duration of time.

Initial studies of hirudin, a naturally occurring direct thrombin inhibitor, yielded promising results. In the HELVETICA trial, 1141 patients who had unstable angina undergoing PCI were randomized to receive intravenous hirudin with or without subcutaneous therapy for 3 days or heparin therapy with the procedure. At 7 days, patients receiving hirudin were significantly less likely to suffer a cardiac event, although this difference was not maintained at 7-month follow-up [120]. In addition, subgroup analysis of two large trials of hirudin as medical therapy for ACS suggested that in those undergoing PCI, hirudin significantly reduced the risk of MI at 30 days compared with heparin. In these same trials, however, it was found that the risk of major bleeding was significantly higher with hirudin [121,122].

Bivalirudin, previously known as hirulog, represents one member in the family of subsequent-generation, synthetic direct thrombin inhibitors. Although other agents in this class have been studied and approved in a variety of noncardiac conditions including heparin-induced thrombocytopenia and venous thromboembolic disease, bivalirudin boasts the most data in the arena of ACS and PCI. Initial use of bivalirudin as a primary anticoagulant in patients who have unstable angina undergoing PTCA was based on the cumulative results from the BAT, CACHET, and REPLACE-1 trials. These trials suggested that bivalirudin reduced major adverse cardiac ischemic events and partially reduced major bleeding complications compared with heparin [123–125]. The potential uncoupling of periprocedural ischemic events and bleeding risk was very encouraging and provided further basis for the REPLACE-2 study. In this large study, 6010 patients undergoing coronary stenting were randomized to receive heparin with planned glycoprotein IIb/IIIa inhibition or bivalirudin with provisional glycoprotein IIb/IIIa inhibitor therapy. Nearly all patients received clopidogrel pretreatment, and only 7% of patients in the bivalirudin arm required provisional glycoprotein IIb/IIIa use, primarily for angiographic complications. Statistically designed to establish noninferiority for the primary end point of death, MI, urgent revascularization, or major in-hospital bleeding, bivalirudin satisfied all prespecified criteria to make this claim. Although there was a nonsignificant reduction in postprocedural non-STEMI in the heparin plus glycoprotein IIb/IIIa inhibitor group compared with the bivalirudin group (5.8% versus 6.6%), this difference did not translate into a mortality benefit at 1-year follow-up. In addition to similar efficacy, bivalirudin was found to be associated with a significant reduction in protocol-defined major bleeding (2.4% versus 4.1%) [126,127].

The increased safety of a PCI anticoagulation strategy using bivalirudin as opposed to UFH may be even greater in patients who have impaired renal function because bivalirudin clearance is comparatively less dependent on renal clearance. A recent pooled analysis of three trials including 5035 patients undergoing PCI evaluated this concept. In this study, the absolute benefit in terms of bleeding and ischemic risk of bivalirudin over heparin was 2.2%, 5.8%, 7.7%, and 14.4%

in patients who had normal, mildly, moderately, or severely reduced renal function, respectively (Fig. 12) [128]. Overall, REPLACE-2, along with various trials preceding it, effectively established bivalirudin as an acceptable alternative to UFH with routine glycoprotein IIb/IIIa inhibition in elective PCI. Especially in patients considered low to moderate risk for periprocedural ischemic complications or high risk for periprocedural bleeding complications, this agent should be strongly considered. The ongoing ACUITY trial is examining the specific role of bivalirudin in high-risk ACS patients managed in an aggressive, contemporary approach, whereas the ongoing HORIZONS trial is evaluating bivalirudin in the setting of primary PCI of STEMI patients [129].

Novel antithrombin agents

The advancement in pharmacotherapy during PCI over the last several years has been impressive. The promise of continued improvements in efficacy and safety exists as next-generation compounds in existing drug classes and entirely new classes of agents continue to be developed. One such class includes the direct factor Xa inhibitors, which by exerting their effect upstream in the coagulation cascade may provide more amplified inhibition of thrombin. Fondaparinux, an existing indirect inhibitor of factor Xa acting by way of antithrombin, showed safety and efficacy in the ASPIRE trial of

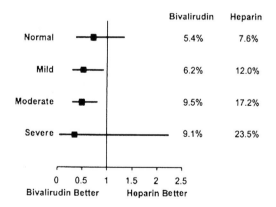

Fig. 12. Odds ratio plots for the quadruple end point of death, MI, urgent revascularization, and major hemorrhage in patients treated with bivalirudin versus heparin, stratified by renal function. (*From* Chew DP, Bhatt DL, Kimball W, et al. Bivalirudin provides increasing benefit with decreasing renal function: a meta-analysis of randomized trials. Am J Cardiol 2003;92(8):919–23; with permission.)

350 patients undergoing urgent or elective PCI [130]. The 20,000-patient OASIS-5 trial of ACS showed favorable ischemic outcomes with fondaparinux versus enoxaparin in ACS, with less bleeding. There was, however, a concern of possibly increased rates of catheter-associated thrombus with fondaparinux [131]. The OASIS-6 trial in patients who have STEMI will provide more information about fondaparinux in PCI. A large number of direct factor Xa inhibitors have been developed, including DX-9065a and otamixaban. XaNADU-ACS, a phase II trial of DX-9065a versus heparin in 402 patients who have ACS in whom glycoprotein IIb/IIIa inhibition and early PCI were encouraged, demonstrated a nonsignificant trend toward improved efficacy and less bleeding [132]. Similarly, XaNADU-PCI evaluated this agent in elective PCI patients and found consistent results with respect to safety and efficacy while providing rationale for the recommended dosing regimen [133]. It does not appear, however, that clinical development of this compound will proceed. SEPIA-PCI, a dose-ranging phase II study of otamixaban versus UFH in nonurgent PCI patients, has completed enrollment. In aggregate, these studies will provide a solid foundation on which larger scale clinical trials of direct factor Xa inhibitors can be performed.

Another major class of novel antithrombotics under current investigation is the TF inhibitors. Exposure of coagulation factors to TF present in the subendothelial layer during the plaque rupture and vessel injury seen with ACS and PCI is a critical step in the subsequent generation of thrombin and the platelet-rich thrombus [134]. Applying the same general concept that upstream coagulation cascade inhibition may lead to amplified anticoagulation, two TF antagonists have currently been developed. Sunol-cH36, a chimeric monoclonal antibody directed against TF, mediates its anticoagulant effect by inhibiting binding of factor X to the TF:VIIa complex, a critical proximal step in the coagulation cascade. PROXIMATE–TIMI 27, the first trial of this agent in humans, evaluated the safety, pharmacokinetics, and dosing of this agent in 26 patients who had stable coronary artery disease. Sunol-cH36 was found to have dose-dependent anticoagulation effects at the cost of only a slight increase in the incidence of minor nonplatelet count–dependent mucosal bleeding [135]. Larger trials of safety and efficacy using this agent are being planned. The other agent in the class of TF inhibitors that is currently being evaluated is the recombinant nematode-associated protein c2 (rNAPc2).

Originally isolated from the hematophageous nematode hookworm, *Anclyostoma caninum*, this agent, like sunol-cH36, also blocks the TF:VIIa enzymatic complex [136]. The recently completed phase IIa dose-confirmation portion of the ANTHEM–TIMI 32 study conducted in 203 patients who had ACS treated with rNAPc2 or placebo in addition to standard antithrombotic therapy demonstrated a dose-related inhibition of thrombin generation. In addition, major and minor bleeding rates were not statistically different between the two treatment groups (4.3% in rNAPc2 group versus 2.5% in placebo group) [137]. The follow-up heparin-replacement portion of this study will further evaluate the efficacy and safety of rNAPc2 by reducing the dose of and ultimately replacing UFH in 50 to 100 patients being treated for ACS.

Summary

The extensive clinical study of antiplatelet and anticoagulant therapy in PCI documented in this review has not only justified the standard of care but also provided the framework for the introduction of novel therapeutic agents such as those discussed previously. Although the evolution to this current standard has been relatively rapid and there have been substantial advancements made in this arena, there remains a clinically relevant rate of ischemic and bleeding complications. This fact, coupled with ongoing advancements in the understanding of mechanisms of vascular injury and thrombosis with ACS and PCI, continues to drive researchers and clinicians to develop new classes of agents with improved pharmacokinetic, efficacy, and safety profiles. Currently, patient- and lesion-specific characteristics guide the interventionalist in deciding which specific antithrombotic and antiplatelet agents to use before, during, and after PCI. In the future, pharmacogenomics, the science of examining genetic variations that dictate response to drug therapy, may play a role in the choice of anticoagulation for any given patient. Until that time, however, the continued execution of well-designed clinical trials of existing and novel pharmacotherapeutic agents and adherence to the findings of such trials is necessary to optimize the outcomes in the growing population of patients undergoing PCI.

Appendix 1. Glossary of clinical trial acronyms

ACE—Abciximab and Carbostent Evaluation trial

ACUITY—Acute Catheterization and Urgent Intervention Triage strategY

ADMIRAL—Abciximab before Direct angioplasty and stenting in Myocardial Infarction Regarding Acute and Long-term follow-up

ADVANCE—ADditive Value of tirofiban Administered with the high-dose bolus in the preventioN of ischemic Complications during high-risk coronary artEry angioplasty

ALBION—Assessment of the best Loading dose of clopidogrel to Blunt platelet activation, Inflammation, and Ongoing Necrosis

ANTHEM—Anticoagulation with Napc2 To Help Eliminate Mace

ARMYDA—Antiplatelet therapy for Reduction of MYocardial Damage during Angioplasty

ASPIRE—Arixtra Study in Percutaneous coronary Intervention: a Randomized Evaluation

BAT—Bivalirudin Angioplasty Trial

CACHET—Comparison of Abciximab Complications with Hirulog ischemic Events Trial

CADILLAC—Controlled Abciximab and Device Investigation to Lower Late Angioplasty Complications

CAPTURE—C7E3 AntiPlatelet Therapy in Unstable REfractory angina

CHARISMA—Clopidogrel for High Atherothrombotic Risk and Ischemic Stabilization, Management and Avoidance

CLASSICS—CLopidogrel ASpirin Stent International Cooperative Study

CREDO—Clopidogrel for the Reduction of Events During Observation

CRUISE—Coronary Revascularization Using Integrilin and Single-bolus Enoxaparin

CURE—Clopidogrel in Unstable angina to prevent Recurrent Events

DISPERSE-2—Dose Confirmation and Feasibility Study of AZD614O + Acetyl Salicylic Acid (ASA) Compared with Clopidogrel + ASA in Patients with Non-ST Segment Elevation Acute Coronary Syndromes

ELECT—EvaLuating Enoxaparin Clotting Times

EPIC—Evaluation of c7E3 for Prevention of Ischemic Complications

EPILOG—Evaluation in PTCA to Improve Long-term Outcome with abciximab Glycoprotein IIb/IIIa blockade

EPISTENT—Evaluation of Platelet IIb/IIIa Inhibitor for STENTing trial

ESPRIT—Enhanced Suppression of the Platelet IIb/IIIa Receptor with Integrilin Therapy

FANTASTIC—Full ANTicoagulation versus ASpirin and TIClopidine

HELVETICA—Hirudin in a European restenosis prevention triaL VErsus heparin Treatment In ptCA patients

HORIZONS—Harmonizing Outcomes with RevascularIZatiON and Stents

IMPACT—Integrilin to Manage Platelet Aggregation to prevent Coronary Thrombosis

INTERACT—INTegrelin and Enoxaparin Randomized assessment of Acute Coronary syndrome Treatment

ISAR–CHOICE—Intracoronary Stenting and Antithrombotic Regimen–Choose between three High Oral doses for Immediate Clopidogrel Effect

ISAR–REACT—Intracoronary Stenting and Antithrombotic Regimen–Rapid Early Action for Coronary Treatment

ISAR–SWEET—Intracoronary Stenting and Antithrombotic Regimen–is abciximab a Superior Way to Eliminate Elevated Thrombotic risk in diabetics

JUMBO–TIMI 26—Joint Use of Medications to Block Platelets Optimally

NICE—National Investigators Collaborating on Enoxaparin

OASIS—Organization to Assess Strategies for Ischemia Syndromes

PARAGON—Platelet IIb/IIIa Antagonism for the Reduction of Acute coronary syndrome events in the Global Organization Network

PRISM–PLUS—Platelet Receptor Inhibition for ischemic Syndrome Management in Patients Limited to very Unstable signs and Symptoms

PROXIMATE—PROXimal Inhibition of coagulation using a Monoclonal Antibody to TissuE factor (Sunol cH36)

PURSUIT—Platelet glycoprotein IIb/IIIa in Unstable angina: Receptor Suppression Using Integrilin Therapy

RAPPORT—ReoPro And Primary PTCA Organization and Randomized Trial

REPLACE—Randomized Evaluation in PCI Linking Angiomax to reduced Clinical Events

RESTORE—Randomized Efficacy Study of Tirofiban for Outcomes and REstenosis

SEPIA–PCI—Study to Evaluate the Pharmacodynamics, the safety and tolerability, and the pharmacokinetics of several Intravenous regimens of the factor XA inhibitor otamixaban, in comparison to intravenous unfractionated heparin, in subjects undergoing nonurgent Percutaneous Coronary Intervention

STARS—STent Anticoagulation Restenosis Study

STEEPLE—SafeTy and Efficacy of Enoxaparin in Percutaneous coronary intervention patients, an internationaL randomized Evaluation

SYNERGY—Superior Yield of the New strategy of Enoxaparin, Revascularization, and GlYcoprotein IIb/IIIa inhibitors

TARGET—do Tirofiban And ReoPro Give similar Efficacy outcomes Trial

TIMI—Thrombolysis In Myocardial Infarction

TRITON–TIMI 38—TRial to assess Improvement in Therapeutic Outcomes by optimizing platelet inhibitioN with prasugrel

XaNADU—First Experience with Direct, Selective Factor XA Inhibition in Patients with Non-ST-elevation Acute Coronary Syndromes

References

[1] Patrono C, Ciabattoni G, Patrignani P, et al. Clinical pharmacology of platelet cyclooxygenase inhibition. Circulation 1985;72(6):1177–84.

[2] Patrignani P, Filabozzi P, Patrono C. Selective cumulative inhibition of platelet thromboxane production by low-dose aspirin in healthy subjects. J Clin Invest 1982;69(6):1366–72.

[3] Barnathan ES, Schwartz JS, Taylor L, et al. Aspirin and dipyridamole in the prevention of acute coronary thrombosis complicating coronary angioplasty. Circulation 1987;76(1):125–34.

[4] Schwartz L, Bourassa MG, Lesperance J, et al. Aspirin and dipyridamole in the prevention of restenosis after percutaneous transluminal coronary angioplasty. N Engl J Med 1988;318(26):1714–9.

[5] Lembo NJ, Black AJ, Roubin GS, et al. Effect of pretreatment with aspirin versus aspirin plus dipyridamole on frequency and type of acute complications of percutaneous transluminal coronary angioplasty. Am J Cardiol 1990;65(7):422–6.

[6] Peters RJ, Mehta SR, Fox KA, et al. Effects of aspirin dose when used alone or in combination with clopidogrel in patients with acute coronary syndromes: observations from the Clopidogrel in Unstable angina to prevent Recurrent Events (CURE) study. Circulation 2003;108(14):1682–7.

[7] Mufson LH. A randomized trial of aspirin in PTCA: effect of high dose versus low dose aspirin on major complications and restenosis. J Am Coll Cardiol 1988;11:236A.

[8] Smith SCJ, Feldman TE, Hirshfeld JW Jr, et al. ACC/AHA/SCAI 2005 guideline update for percutaneous coronary intervention—summary article: a report of the American College of Cardiology/American Heart Association Task Force on Practice Guidelines (ACC/AHA/SCAI Writing Committee to Update the 2001 Guidelines for Percutaneous Coronary Intervention). Circulation 2006;113:1–20.

[9] Mason PJ, Jacobs AK, Freedman JE. Aspirin resistance and atherothrombotic disease. J Am Coll Cardiol 2005;46(6):986–93.

[10] Gum PA, Kottke-Marchant K, Welsh PA, et al. A prospective, blinded determination of the natural history of aspirin resistance among stable patients with cardiovascular disease. J Am Coll Cardiol 2003;41(6):961–5.

[11] Sharis PJ, Cannon CP, Loscalzo J. The antiplatelet effects of ticlopidine and clopidogrel. Ann Intern Med 1998;129(5):394–405.

[12] Altmann DB, Racz M, Battleman DS, et al. Reduction in angioplasty complications after the introduction of coronary stents: results from a consecutive series of 2242 patients. Am Heart J 1996;132(3):503–7.

[13] Leon MB, Baim DS, Popma JJ, et al. A clinical trial comparing three antithrombotic-drug regimens after coronary-artery stenting. Stent Anticoagulation Restenosis Study Investigators. N Engl J Med 1998;339(23):1665–71.

[14] Bertrand ME, Legrand V, Boland J, et al. Randomized multicenter comparison of conventional anticoagulation versus antiplatelet therapy in unplanned and elective coronary stenting. The full anticoagulation versus aspirin and ticlopidine (FANTASTIC) study. Circulation 1998;98(16):1597–603.

[15] Schomig A, Neumann FJ, Kastrati A, et al. A randomized comparison of antiplatelet and anticoagulant therapy after the placement of coronary-artery stents. N Engl J Med 1996;334(17):1084–9.

[16] Schomig A, Neumann FJ, Walter H, et al. Coronary stent placement in patients with acute myocardial infarction: comparison of clinical and angiographic outcome after randomization to antiplatelet or anticoagulant therapy. J Am Coll Cardiol 1997;29(1):28–34.

[17] Urban P, Macaya C, Rupprecht HJ, et al. Randomized evaluation of anticoagulation versus antiplatelet therapy after coronary stent implantation in high-risk patients: the Multicenter Aspirin and Ticlopidine Trial after Intracoronary Stenting (MATTIS). Circulation 1998;98(20):2126–32.

[18] Neumann FJ, Hall D, Schomig A. Neutropenia with ticlopidine plus aspirin. Lancet 1997;349(9064):1552–3.

[19] Steinhubl SR, Tan WA, Foody JM, et al. Incidence and clinical course of thrombotic thrombocytopenic purpura due to ticlopidine following coronary stenting. EPISTENT Investigators. Evaluation of Platelet IIb/IIIa Inhibitor for Stenting. JAMA 1999;281(9):806–10.

[20] Bennett CL, Davidson CJ, Raisch DW, et al. Thrombotic thrombocytopenic purpura associated with ticlopidine in the setting of coronary artery stents and stroke prevention. Arch Intern Med 1999;159(21):2524–8.

[21] Bertrand ME, Rupprecht HJ, Urban P, et al. Double-blind study of the safety of clopidogrel with and without a loading dose in combination with aspirin compared with ticlopidine in combination with aspirin after coronary stenting: the Clopidogrel Aspirin Stent International Cooperative Study (CLASSICS). Circulation 2000;102(6):624–9.

[22] Bhatt DL, Bertrand ME, Berger PB, et al. Meta-analysis of randomized and registry comparisons of ticlopidine with clopidogrel after stenting. J Am Coll Cardiol 2002;39(1):9–14.

[23] Quinn MJ, Fitzgerald DJ. Ticlopidine and clopidogrel. Circulation 1999;100(15):1667–72.

[24] Yusuf S, Zhao F, Mehta SR, et al. Effects of clopidogrel in addition to aspirin in patients with acute coronary syndromes without ST-segment elevation. N Engl J Med 2001;345(7):494–502.

[25] Mehta SR, Yusuf S, Peters RJ, et al. Effects of pretreatment with clopidogrel and aspirin followed by long-term therapy in patients undergoing percutaneous coronary intervention: the PCI-CURE study. Lancet 2001;358(9281):527–33.

[26] Steinhubl SR, Berger PB, Mann JT, et al. Early and sustained dual oral antiplatelet therapy following percutaneous coronary intervention: a randomized controlled trial. JAMA 2002;288(19):2411–20.

[27] Muller I, Seyfarth M, Rudiger S, et al. Effect of a high loading dose of clopidogrel on platelet function in patients undergoing coronary stent placement. Heart 2001;85(1):92–3.

[28] Kandzari DE, Berger PB, Kastrati A, et al. Influence of treatment duration with a 600-mg dose of clopidogrel before percutaneous coronary revascularization. J Am Coll Cardiol 2004;44(11):2133–6.

[29] Patti G, Colonna G, Pasceri V, et al. Randomized trial of high loading dose of clopidogrel for reduction of periprocedural myocardial infarction in patients undergoing coronary intervention: results from the ARMYDA-2 (Antiplatelet therapy for Reduction of MYocardial Damage during Angioplasty) study. Circulation 2005;111(16):2099–106.

[30] Montalescot G. Assessment of the Best Loading Dose of Clopidogrel to Blunt Platelet Activation, Inflammation, and Ongoing Necrosis (ALBION) trial. Presented at the 12th EuroPCR. Paris, France, May 24–27, 2005.

[31] von Beckerath N, Taubert D, Pogatsa-Murray G, et al. Absorption, metabolization, and antiplatelet effects of 300-, 600-, and 900-mg loading doses of clopidogrel: results of the ISAR-CHOICE (Intracoronary Stenting and Antithrombotic Regimen: Choose Between 3 High Oral Doses for Immediate Clopidogrel Effect) trial. Circulation 2005;112(19):2946–50.

[32] Moreno R, Fernandez C, Hernandez R, et al. Drug-eluting stent thrombosis: results from a pooled analysis including 10 randomized studies. J Am Coll Cardiol 2005;45(6):954–9.

[33] Nguyen TA, Diodati JG, Pharand C. Resistance to clopidogrel: a review of the evidence. J Am Coll Cardiol 2005;45(8):1157–64.

[34] Niitsu Y, Jakubowski JA, Sugidachi A, et al. Pharmacology of CS-747 (prasugrel, LY640315), a novel, potent antiplatelet agent with in vivo P2Y12 receptor antagonist activity. Semin Thromb Hemost 2005;31(2):184–94.

[35] Wiviott SD, Antman EM, Winters KJ, et al. Randomized comparison of prasugrel (CS-747, LY640315), a novel thienopyridine P2Y12 antagonist, with clopidogrel in percutaneous coronary intervention: results of the Joint Utilization of Medications to Block Platelets Optimally (JUMBO)-TIMI 26 trial. Circulation 2005;111(25):3366–73.

[36] van Giezen JJ, Humphries RG. Preclinical and clinical studies with selective reversible direct P2Y12 antagonists. Semin Thromb Hemost 2005;31(2):195–204.

[37] Cannon CP. The DISPERSE 2 trial: safety, tolerability, and preliminary efficacy of AZD6140, the first oral, reversible ADP receptor antagonist, compared with clopidogrel in patients with non-ST segment elevation acute coronary syndrome. Presented at the 51st American Heart Association Scientific Sessions. Dallas (TX), November 13–16, 2005.

[38] Bhatt DL, Topol EJ. Clopidogrel added to aspirin versus aspirin alone in secondary prevention and high-risk primary prevention: rationale and design of the Clopidogrel for High Atherothrombotic Risk and Ischemic Stabilization, Management, and Avoidance (CHARISMA) trial. Am Heart J 2004;148(2):263–8.

[39] Hynes RO. Integrins: a family of cell surface receptors. Cell 1987;48(4):549–54.

[40] Plow EF, Ginsberg MH. Cellular adhesion: GPIIb-IIIa as a prototypic adhesion receptor. Prog Hemost Thromb 1989;9:117–56.

[41] Coller BS. A new murine monoclonal antibody reports an activation-dependent change in the conformation and/or microenvironment of the platelet glycoprotein IIb/IIIa complex. J Clin Invest 1985;76(1):101–8.

[42] Coller BS, Scudder LE. Inhibition of dog platelet function by in vivo infusion of F(ab')2 fragments of a monoclonal antibody to the platelet glycoprotein IIb/IIIa receptor. Blood 1985;66(6):1456–9.

[43] Ellis SG, Tcheng JE, Navetta FI, et al. Safety and antiplatelet effect of murine monoclonal antibody

7E3 Fab directed against platelet glycoprotein IIb/IIIa in patients undergoing elective coronary angioplasty. Coron Artery Dis 1993;4(2):167–75.

[44] Use of a monoclonal antibody directed against the platelet glycoprotein IIb/IIIa receptor in high-risk coronary angioplasty. The EPIC Investigation. N Engl J Med 1994;330(14):956–61.

[45] Topol EJ, Ferguson JJ, Weisman HF, et al. Long-term protection from myocardial ischemic events in a randomized trial of brief integrin beta3 blockade with percutaneous coronary intervention. EPIC Investigator Group. Evaluation of Platelet IIb/IIIa Inhibition for Prevention of Ischemic Complication. JAMA 1997;278(6):479–84.

[46] Platelet glycoprotein IIb/IIIa receptor blockade and low-dose heparin during percutaneous coronary revascularization. The EPILOG Investigators. N Engl J Med 1997;336(24):1689–96.

[47] Lincoff AM, Tcheng JE, Califf RM, et al. Sustained suppression of ischemic complications of coronary intervention by platelet GP IIb/IIIa blockade with abciximab: one-year outcome in the EPILOG trial. Evaluation in PTCA to Improve Long-term Outcome with abciximab GP IIb/IIIa blockade. Circulation 1999;99(15):1951–8.

[48] Randomised placebo-controlled and balloon-angioplasty-controlled trial to assess safety of coronary stenting with use of platelet glycoprotein-IIb/IIIa blockade. The EPISTENT Investigators. Evaluation of Platelet IIb/IIIa Inhibitor for Stenting. Lancet 1998;352(9122):87–92.

[49] Lincoff AM, Califf RM, Moliterno DJ, et al. Complementary clinical benefits of coronary-artery stenting and blockade of platelet glycoprotein IIb/IIIa receptors. Evaluation of Platelet IIb/IIIa Inhibition in Stenting Investigators. N Engl J Med 1999;341(5):319–27.

[50] Topol EJ, Mark DB, Lincoff AM, et al. Outcomes at 1 year and economic implications of platelet glycoprotein IIb/IIIa blockade in patients undergoing coronary stenting: results from a multicentre randomised trial. EPISTENT Investigators. Evaluation of Platelet IIb/IIIa Inhibitor for Stenting. Lancet 1999;354(9195):2019–24.

[51] Cho L, Topol EJ, Balog C, et al. Clinical benefit of glycoprotein IIb/IIIa blockade with abciximab is independent of gender: pooled analysis from EPIC, EPILOG and EPISTENT trials. Evaluation of 7E3 for the Prevention of Ischemic Complications. Evaluation in Percutaneous Transluminal Coronary Angioplasty to Improve Long-Term Outcome with Abciximab GP IIb/IIIa blockade. Evaluation of Platelet IIb/IIIa Inhibitor for Stenting. J Am Coll Cardiol 2000;36(2):381–6.

[52] Topol EJ, Lincoff AM, Kereiakes DJ, et al. Multi-year follow-up of abciximab therapy in three randomized, placebo-controlled trials of percutaneous coronary revascularization. Am J Med 2002;113(1):1–6.

[53] Randomised placebo-controlled trial of abciximab before and during coronary intervention in refractory unstable angina: the CAPTURE Study. Lancet 1997;349(9063):1429–35.

[54] Cura FA, Bhatt DL, Lincoff AM, et al. Pronounced benefit of coronary stenting and adjunctive platelet glycoprotein IIb/IIIa inhibition in complex atherosclerotic lesions. Circulation 2000;102(1):28–34.

[55] Bhatt DL, Marso SP, Lincoff AM, et al. Abciximab reduces mortality in diabetics following percutaneous coronary intervention. J Am Coll Cardiol 2000;35(4):922–8.

[56] Mehilli J, Kastrati A, Schuhlen H, et al. Randomized clinical trial of abciximab in diabetic patients undergoing elective percutaneous coronary interventions after treatment with a high loading dose of clopidogrel. Circulation 2004;110(24):3627–35.

[57] Tam SH, Sassoli PM, Jordan RE, et al. Abciximab (ReoPro, chimeric 7E3 Fab) demonstrates equivalent affinity and functional blockade of glycoprotein IIb/IIIa and alpha(v)beta3 integrins. Circulation 1998;98(11):1085–91.

[58] Acute platelet inhibition with abciximab does not reduce in-stent restenosis (ERASER study). The ERASER Investigators. Circulation 1999;100(8):799–806.

[59] Montalescot G, Barragan P, Wittenberg O, et al. Platelet glycoprotein IIb/IIIa inhibition with coronary stenting for acute myocardial infarction. N Engl J Med 2001;344(25):1895–903.

[60] Montalescot G, Borentain M, Payot L, et al. Early vs late administration of glycoprotein IIb/IIIa inhibitors in primary percutaneous coronary intervention of acute ST-segment elevation myocardial infarction: a meta-analysis. JAMA 2004;292(3):362–6.

[61] Three-year duration of benefit from abciximab in patients receiving stents for acute myocardial infarction in the randomized double-blind ADMIRAL study. Eur Heart J 2005;26(23):2520–3.

[62] Neumann FJ, Kastrati A, Schmitt C, et al. Effect of glycoprotein IIb/IIIa receptor blockade with abciximab on clinical and angiographic restenosis rate after the placement of coronary stents following acute myocardial infarction. J Am Coll Cardiol 2000;35(4):915–21.

[63] Brener SJ, Barr LA, Burchenal JE, et al. Randomized, placebo-controlled trial of platelet glycoprotein IIb/IIIa blockade with primary angioplasty for acute myocardial infarction. ReoPro And Primary PTCA Organization and Randomized Trial (RAPPORT) Investigators. Circulation 1998;98(8):734–41.

[64] Antoniucci D, Rodriguez A, Hempel A, et al. A randomized trial comparing primary infarct artery stenting with or without abciximab in acute myocardial infarction. J Am Coll Cardiol 2003;42(11):1879–85.

[65] Antoniucci D, Migliorini A, Parodi G, et al. Abciximab-supported infarct artery stent implantation for acute myocardial infarction and long-term survival: a prospective, multicenter, randomized trial comparing infarct artery stenting plus abciximab with stenting alone. Circulation 2004;109(14): 1704–6.

[66] Stone GW, Grines CL, Cox DA, et al. Comparison of angioplasty with stenting, with or without abciximab, in acute myocardial infarction. N Engl J Med 2002;346(13):957–66.

[67] De Luca G, Suryapranata H, Stone GW, et al. Abciximab as adjunctive therapy to reperfusion in acute ST-segment elevation myocardial infarction: a meta-analysis of randomized trials. JAMA 2005;293(14):1759–65.

[68] Phillips DR, Scarborough RM. Clinical pharmacology of eptifibatide. Am J Cardiol 1997;80(4A): 11B–20B.

[69] Harrington RA, Kleiman NS, Kottke-Marchant K, et al. Immediate and reversible platelet inhibition after intravenous administration of a peptide glycoprotein IIb/IIIa inhibitor during percutaneous coronary intervention. Am J Cardiol 1995; 76(17):1222–7.

[70] Inhibition of platelet glycoprotein IIb/IIIa with eptifibatide in patients with acute coronary syndromes. The PURSUIT Trial Investigators. Platelet Glycoprotein IIb/IIIa in Unstable Angina: Receptor Suppression Using Integrilin Therapy. N Engl J Med 1998;339(7):436–43.

[71] Kleiman NS, Lincoff AM, Flaker GC, et al. Early percutaneous coronary intervention, platelet inhibition with eptifibatide, and clinical outcomes in patients with acute coronary syndromes. PURSUIT Investigators. Circulation 2000;101(7): 751–7.

[72] Randomised placebo-controlled trial of effect of eptifibatide on complications of percutaneous coronary intervention: IMPACT-II. Integrilin to Minimise Platelet Aggregation and Coronary Thrombosis-II. Lancet 1997;349(9063):1422–8.

[73] Phillips DR, Teng W, Arfsten A, et al. Effect of Ca2 + on GP IIb-IIIa interactions with integrilin: enhanced GP IIb-IIIa binding and inhibition of platelet aggregation by reductions in the concentration of ionized calcium in plasma anticoagulated with citrate. Circulation 1997;96(5):1488–94.

[74] Tcheng JE, Talley JD, O'Shea JC, et al. Clinical pharmacology of higher dose eptifibatide in percutaneous coronary intervention (the PRIDE study). Am J Cardiol 2001;88(10):1097–102.

[75] Novel dosing regimen of eptifibatide in planned coronary stent implantation (ESPRIT): a randomised, placebo-controlled trial. Lancet 2000; 356(9247):2037–44.

[76] O'Shea JC, Hafley GE, Greenberg S, et al. Platelet glycoprotein IIb/IIIa integrin blockade with eptifibatide in coronary stent intervention: the ESPRIT trial: a randomized controlled trial. JAMA 2001; 285(19):2468–73.

[77] O'Shea JC, Buller CE, Cantor WJ, et al. Long-term efficacy of platelet glycoprotein IIb/IIIa integrin blockade with eptifibatide in coronary stent intervention. JAMA 2002;287(5):618–21.

[78] Dasgupta H, Blankenship JC, Wood GC, et al. Thrombocytopenia complicating treatment with intravenous glycoprotein IIb/IIIa receptor inhibitors: a pooled analysis. Am Heart J 2000;140(2): 206–11.

[79] Kereiakes DJ, Kleiman NS, Ambrose J, et al. Randomized, double-blind, placebo-controlled dose-ranging study of tirofiban (MK-383) platelet IIb/IIIa blockade in high risk patients undergoing coronary angioplasty. J Am Coll Cardiol 1996;27(3): 536–42.

[80] Effects of platelet glycoprotein IIb/IIIa blockade with tirofiban on adverse cardiac events in patients with unstable angina or acute myocardial infarction undergoing coronary angioplasty. The RESTORE Investigators. Randomized Efficacy Study of Tirofiban for Outcomes and REstenosis. Circulation 1997;96(5):1445–53.

[81] Gibson CM, Goel M, Cohen DJ, et al. Six-month angiographic and clinical follow-up of patients prospectively randomized to receive either tirofiban or placebo during angioplasty in the RESTORE trial. Randomized Efficacy Study of Tirofiban for Outcomes and Restenosis. J Am Coll Cardiol 1998; 32(1):28–34.

[82] Inhibition of the platelet glycoprotein IIb/IIIa receptor with tirofiban in unstable angina and non-Q-wave myocardial infarction. Platelet Receptor Inhibition in Ischemic Syndrome Management in Patients Limited by Unstable Signs and Symptoms (PRISM-PLUS) Study Investigators. N Engl J Med 1998;338(21):1488–97.

[83] Sabatine MS, Januzzi JL, Snapinn S, et al. A risk score system for predicting adverse outcomes and magnitude of benefit with glycoprotein IIb/IIIa inhibitor therapy in patients with unstable angina pectoris. Am J Cardiol 2001;88(5):488–92.

[84] Valgimigli M, Percoco G, Barbieri D, et al. The additive value of tirofiban administered with the high-dose bolus in the prevention of ischemic complications during high-risk coronary angioplasty: the ADVANCE Trial. J Am Coll Cardiol 2004; 44(1):14–9.

[85] Roffi M, Mukherjee D, Chew DP, et al. Lack of benefit from intravenous platelet glycoprotein IIb/IIIa receptor inhibition as adjunctive treatment for percutaneous interventions of aortocoronary bypass grafts: a pooled analysis of five randomized clinical trials. Circulation 2002;106(24):3063–7.

[86] Karvouni E, Katritsis DG, Ioannidis JP. Intravenous glycoprotein IIb/IIIa receptor antagonists reduce mortality after percutaneous coronary interventions. J Am Coll Cardiol 2003;41(1):26–32.

[87] Boersma E, Harrington RA, Moliterno DJ, et al. Platelet glycoprotein IIb/IIIa inhibitors in acute coronary syndromes: a meta-analysis of all major randomised clinical trials. Lancet 2002;359(9302): 189–98.

[88] Roffi M, Chew DP, Mukherjee D, et al. Platelet glycoprotein IIb/IIIa inhibitors reduce mortality in diabetic patients with non-ST-segment-elevation acute coronary syndromes. Circulation 2001;104(23): 2767–71.

[89] Brown DL, Fann CS, Chang CJ. Meta-analysis of effectiveness and safety of abciximab versus eptifibatide or tirofiban in percutaneous coronary intervention. Am J Cardiol 2001;87(5):537–41.

[90] Topol EJ, Moliterno DJ, Herrmann HC, et al. Comparison of two platelet glycoprotein IIb/IIIa inhibitors, tirofiban and abciximab, for the prevention of ischemic events with percutaneous coronary revascularization. N Engl J Med 2001;344(25): 1888–94.

[91] Theroux P, Kouz S, Roy L, et al. Platelet membrane receptor glycoprotein IIb/IIIa antagonism in unstable angina. The Canadian Lamifiban Study. Circulation 1996;94(5):899–905.

[92] International randomized, controlled trial of lamifiban (a platelet glycoprotein IIb/IIIa inhibitor), heparin, or both in unstable angina. The PARAGON Investigators. Platelet IIb/IIIa Antagonism for the Reduction of Acute coronary syndrome events in a Global Organization Network. Circulation 1998;97(24):2386–95.

[93] Randomized placebo-controlled trial of titrated intravenous lamifiban for acute coronary syndromes. Circulation 2002;105(3):316–21.

[94] Chew DP, Bhatt DL, Sapp S, et al. Increased mortality with oral platelet glycoprotein IIb/IIIa antagonists: a meta-analysis of phase III multicenter randomized trials. Circulation 2001;103(2):201–6.

[95] Hirsh J, Warkentin TE, Shaughnessy SG, et al. Heparin and low-molecular-weight heparin: mechanisms of action, pharmacokinetics, dosing, monitoring, efficacy, and safety. Chest 2001; 119(1 Suppl):64S–94S.

[96] Chew DP, Bhatt DL, Lincoff AM, et al. Defining the optimal activated clotting time during percutaneous coronary intervention: aggregate results from 6 randomized, controlled trials. Circulation 2001;103(7):961–6.

[97] Brener SJ, Moliterno DJ, Lincoff AM, et al. Relationship between activated clotting time and ischemic or hemorrhagic complications: analysis of 4 recent randomized clinical trials of percutaneous coronary intervention. Circulation 2004;110(8): 994–8.

[98] Ferguson JJ, Dohmen P, Wilson JM, et al. Results of a national survey on anticoagulation for PTCA. J Invasive Cardiol 1995;7(5):136–41.

[99] Rabah M, Mason D, Muller DW, et al. Heparin after percutaneous intervention (HAPI): a prospective multicenter randomized trial of three heparin regimens after successful coronary intervention. J Am Coll Cardiol 1999;34(2):461–7.

[100] Hirsh J, Raschke R. Heparin and low-molecular-weight heparin: the Seventh ACCP Conference on Antithrombotic and Thrombolytic Therapy. Chest 2004;126(3 Suppl):188S–203S.

[101] Warkentin TE, Greinacher A. Heparin-induced thrombocytopenia: recognition, treatment, and prevention: the Seventh ACCP Conference on Antithrombotic and Thrombolytic Therapy. Chest 2004;126(3 Suppl):311S–37S.

[102] Rabah MM, Premmereur J, Graham M, et al. Usefulness of intravenous enoxaparin for percutaneous coronary intervention in stable angina pectoris. Am J Cardiol 1999;84(12):1391–5.

[103] Young JJ, Kereiakes DJ, Grines CL. Low-molecular-weight heparin therapy in percutaneous coronary intervention: the NICE 1 and NICE 4 trials. National Investigators Collaborating on Enoxaparin Investigators. J Invasive Cardiol 2000; 12(Suppl E):E14–8 [discussion: E25–8].

[104] Kereiakes DJ, Grines C, Fry E, et al. Enoxaparin and abciximab adjunctive pharmacotherapy during percutaneous coronary intervention. J Invasive Cardiol 2001;13(4):272–8.

[105] Bhatt DL, Lee BI, Casterella PJ, et al. Safety of concomitant therapy with eptifibatide and enoxaparin in patients undergoing percutaneous coronary intervention: results of the Coronary Revascularization Using Integrilin and Single bolus Enoxaparin Study. J Am Coll Cardiol 2003; 41(1):20–5.

[106] Montalescot G. STEEPLE: Safety and Efficacy of Enoxaparin in Percutaneous Coronary Intervention Patients, an International Randomized Evaluation. Presented at the 27th European Society of Cardiology Congress. Stockholm, Sweden, September 3–7, 2005.

[107] Cohen M, Demers C, Gurfinkel EP, et al. A comparison of low-molecular-weight heparin with unfractionated heparin for unstable coronary artery disease. Efficacy and Safety of Subcutaneous Enoxaparin in Non-Q-Wave Coronary Events Study Group. N Engl J Med 1997;337(7):447–52.

[108] Antman EM, McCabe CH, Gurfinkel EP, et al. Enoxaparin prevents death and cardiac ischemic events in unstable angina/non-Q-wave myocardial infarction. Results of the Thrombolysis In Myocardial Infarction (TIMI) 11B trial. Circulation 1999; 100(15):1593–601.

[109] Ferguson JJ, Antman EM, Bates ER, et al. Combining enoxaparin and glycoprotein IIb/IIIa antagonists for the treatment of acute coronary syndromes: final results of the National Investigators Collaborating on Enoxaparin-3 (NICE-3) study. Am Heart J 2003;146(4):628–34.

[110] Goodman SG, Fitchett D, Armstrong PW, et al. Randomized evaluation of the safety and efficacy of enoxaparin versus unfractionated heparin in

high-risk patients with non-ST-segment elevation acute coronary syndromes receiving the glycoprotein IIb/IIIa inhibitor eptifibatide. Circulation 2003;107(2):238–44.

[111] Faxon DP, Spiro TE, Minor S, et al. Low molecular weight heparin in prevention of restenosis after angioplasty. Results of Enoxaparin Restenosis (ERA) Trial. Circulation 1994;90(2):908–14.

[112] Cairns JA, Gill J, Morton B, et al. Fish oils and low-molecular-weight heparin for the reduction of restenosis after percutaneous transluminal coronary angioplasty. The EMPAR Study. Circulation 1996;94(7):1553–60.

[113] Grassman ED, Leya F, Fareed J, et al. A randomized trial of the low-molecular-weight heparin certoparin to prevent restenosis following coronary angioplasty. J Invasive Cardiol 2001;13(11):723–8.

[114] Zidar JP. Low-molecular-weight heparins in coronary stenting (the ENTICES trial). ENoxaparin and TIClopidine after Elective Stenting. Am J Cardiol 1998;82(5B):29L–32L.

[115] Batchelor WB, Mahaffey KW, Berger PB, et al. A randomized, placebo-controlled trial of enoxaparin after high-risk coronary stenting: the ATLAST trial. J Am Coll Cardiol 2001;38(6):1608–13.

[116] Moliterno DJ, Hermiller JB, Kereiakes DJ, et al. A novel point-of-care enoxaparin monitor for use during percutaneous coronary intervention. Results of the Evaluating Enoxaparin Clotting Times (ELECT) Study. J Am Coll Cardiol 2003;42(6):1132–9.

[117] Ferguson JJ, Califf RM, Antman EM, et al. Enoxaparin vs unfractionated heparin in high-risk patients with non-ST-segment elevation acute coronary syndromes managed with an intended early invasive strategy: primary results of the SYNERGY randomized trial. JAMA 2004;292(1):45–54.

[118] Weitz JI, Hudoba M, Massel D, et al. Clot-bound thrombin is protected from inhibition by heparin-antithrombin III but is susceptible to inactivation by antithrombin III-independent inhibitors. J Clin Invest 1990;86(2):385–91.

[119] Eitzman DT, Chi L, Saggin L, et al. Heparin neutralization by platelet-rich thrombi. Role of platelet factor 4. Circulation 1994;89(4):1523–9.

[120] Serruys PW, Herrman JP, Simon R, et al. A comparison of hirudin with heparin in the prevention of restenosis after coronary angioplasty. HELVETICA Investigators. N Engl J Med 1995;333(12):757–63.

[121] Mehta SR, Eikelboom JW, Rupprecht HJ, et al. Efficacy of hirudin in reducing cardiovascular events in patients with acute coronary syndrome undergoing early percutaneous coronary intervention. Eur Heart J 2002;23(2):117–23.

[122] Roe MT, Granger CB, Puma JA, et al. Comparison of benefits and complications of hirudin versus heparin for patients with acute coronary syndromes undergoing early percutaneous coronary intervention. Am J Cardiol 2001;88(12):1403–6, A6.

[123] Bittl JA, Strony J, Brinker JA, et al. Treatment with bivalirudin (Hirulog) as compared with heparin during coronary angioplasty for unstable or postinfarction angina. Hirulog Angioplasty Study Investigators. N Engl J Med 1995;333(12):764–9.

[124] Lincoff AM, Kleiman NS, Kottke-Marchant K, et al. Bivalirudin with planned or provisional abciximab versus low-dose heparin and abciximab during percutaneous coronary revascularization: results of the Comparison of Abciximab Complications with Hirulog for Ischemic Events Trial (CACHET). Am Heart J 2002;143(5):847–53.

[125] Lincoff AM, Bittl JA, Kleiman NS, et al. Comparison of bivalirudin versus heparin during percutaneous coronary intervention (the Randomized Evaluation of PCI Linking Angiomax to Reduced Clinical Events [REPLACE]-1 trial). Am J Cardiol 2004;93(9):1092–6.

[126] Lincoff AM, Bittl JA, Harrington RA, et al. Bivalirudin and provisional glycoprotein IIb/IIIa blockade compared with heparin and planned glycoprotein IIb/IIIa blockade during percutaneous coronary intervention: REPLACE-2 randomized trial. JAMA 2003;289(7):853–63.

[127] Lincoff AM, Kleiman NS, Kereiakes DJ, et al. Long-term efficacy of bivalirudin and provisional glycoprotein IIb/IIIa blockade vs heparin and planned glycoprotein IIb/IIIa blockade during percutaneous coronary revascularization: REPLACE-2 randomized trial. JAMA 2004;292(6):696–703.

[128] Chew DP, Bhatt DL, Kimball W, et al. Bivalirudin provides increasing benefit with decreasing renal function: a meta-analysis of randomized trials. Am J Cardiol 2003;92(8):919–23.

[129] Stone GW, Bertrand M, Colombo A, et al. Acute Catheterization and Urgent Intervention Triage strategY (ACUITY) trial: study design and rationale. Am Heart J 2004;148(5):764–75.

[130] Mehta SR, Steg PG, Granger CB, et al. Randomized, blinded trial comparing fondaparinux with unfractionated heparin in patients undergoing contemporary percutaneous coronary intervention: Arixtra Study in Percutaneous Coronary Intervention: a Randomized Evaluation (ASPIRE) Pilot Trial. Circulation 2005;111(11):1390–7.

[131] Yusuf S. An international, randomized, double-blind study evaluating the efficacy and safety of fondaparinux versus enoxaparin in the acute treatment of unstable angina/non ST-segment elevation MI acute coronary syndromes. Presented at the 27th European Society of Cardiology Congress. Stockholm, Sweden, September 3–7, 2005.

[132] Alexander JH, Yang H, Becker RC, et al. First experience with direct, selective factor Xa inhibition in patients with non-ST-elevation acute coronary syndromes: results of the XaNADU-ACS Trial. J Thromb Haemost 2005;3(3):439–47.

[133] Alexander JH, Dyke CK, Yang H, et al. Initial experience with factor-Xa inhibition in percutaneous coronary intervention: the XaNADU-PCI Pilot. J Thromb Haemost 2004;2(2):234–41.

[134] Toschi V, Gallo R, Lettino M, et al. Tissue factor modulates the thrombogenicity of human atherosclerotic plaques. Circulation 1997;95(3):594–9.

[135] Morrow DA, Murphy SA, McCabe CH, et al. Potent inhibition of thrombin with a monoclonal antibody against tissue factor (Sunol-cH36): results of the PROXIMATE-TIMI 27 trial. Eur Heart J 2005;26(7):682–8.

[136] Stassens P, Bergum PW, Gansemans Y, et al. Anticoagulant repertoire of the hookworm *Ancylostoma caninum*. Proc Natl Acad Sci U S A 1996;93(5): 2149–54.

[137] Giugliano RP, Wiviott SD, Morrow DA, et al. Addition of a tissue-factor/factor VIIa inhibitor to standard treatments in nste-acs managed with an early invasive strategy: results of the phase 2 ANTHEM-TIMI 32 double-blind randomized clinical trial. Presented at the 51st American Heart Association Scientific Sessions. Dallas (TX), November 13–6, 2005.

ELSEVIER
SAUNDERS

Cardiol Clin 24 (2006) 201–215

CARDIOLOGY
CLINICS

Coronary Interventional Devices: Balloon, Atherectomy, Thrombectomy and Distal Protection Devices

Samin K. Sharma, MD, FACC*, Victor Chen, MBChB, FRACP

*Cardiac Catheterization Laboratory, Cardiovascular Institute, Mount Sinai Hospital,
Box 1030, One Gustave Levy Place, New York, NY 10029, USA*

Atherosclerosis is a complex disease in which cholesterol deposition, inflammation, calcification, and thrombus formation play major roles. Rupture of high-risk vulnerable plaques rich in cholesterol and plaque erosion are responsible for occlusive coronary thrombosis and acute coronary events by exposing highly thrombogenic, cholesterol-rich material to the bloodstream. Platelet adhesion and aggregation and activation of the coagulation cascade are induced, which results in thrombus formation. Newly formed thrombus may further impair blood flow and a spectrum of syndromes may ensue, from being minimal or asymptomatic to causing accelerated or unstable angina pectoris, myocardial infarction (acute coronary syndrome [ACS]), or even sudden death. Treatment of coronary or graft lesions with associated thrombus (suspected or angiographically evident) is challenging for an interventionalist, because interventions in these cases are associated with an increased incidence of procedural complications (distal embolization, abrupt occlusion, slow or no-reflow, need for emergent bypass surgery, and death). As an attempt to decrease complications, strategies for removing thrombus from the vessel before and during the percutaneous intervention are developed (eg, thrombectomy and distal protection devices). In other cases atherosclerotic plaque is chronic and bulky, with a high fibrous and calcium content making it resistant to routine dilatation and expansion by balloons or stents. These hard and complex lesions must be modified by debulking and plaque modification adjunctive devices (eg, percutaneous transluminal coronary angioplasty (PTCA), atherectomy, atherotomy, and laser) before stenting to attain good acute results with low complications, decreased rates of stent thrombosis, and perhaps lower restenosis.

Although coronary stent implantation remains the mainstay and ultimate step for percutaneous treatment of most coronary lesions, some adjunctive devices may be required for lesion preparation to facilitate stent deployment and optimal expansion and prevent distal embolization [1,2].

Atherectomy, atherotomy, laser, and other debulking devices

With increased operator experience and improved device technology there has been a constant growth in the number of complex lesions (ie, diffuse lesions, calcified lesions, nondilatable rigid lesions, ostial lesions, bifurcations, and chronic total occlusions) attempted by interventionalists with use of drug-eluting stents (DES), despite the fact that data are lacking in their effectiveness. Procedural complexity, in-hospital complications, and long-term outcome remain major concerns of DES in these complex lesions because of large or resistant plaque burdens leading to stent underexpansion, which possibly increases the chances of stent thrombosis and restenosis. Stent deployment is sometimes difficult in such complex calcified lesions and is prone to problems such as stent entrapment, stent stripping, underexpansion, and

---

* Corresponding author.
E-mail address: samin.sharma@msnyuhealth.org
(S.K. Sharma).

balloon rupture, with attendant risks of major coronary dissection and acute in-hospital complications. Optimal stent expansion and final minimal lumen diameter remain important predictors of restenosis even after DES implantation [3]. Uniform rather than nonuniform stent expansion guarantees the homogenous drug delivery and diffusion into the lesion by maintaining adequate distance between stent struts [4]. Pretreatment of complex lesions with high-pressure noncompliant balloon inflation before DES is an option but is not always successful and may be limited by plaque rigidity, plaque shift, snow plough into side branch, extensive vessel dissection, and even vessel perforation. Incomplete stent apposition has been reported to be a predictor for late stent thrombosis with DES. On the other hand, high-pressure coronary stent implantation in postmortem histopathologic studies has been shown to cause arterial medial disruption, break in internal elastic lamina, or lipid core penetration by stent struts and may induce increased arterial inflammation associated with increased neointimal growth (Fig. 1) [5].

Studies using intravascular ultrasound (IVUS) have suggested that neointimal area was predicted by the degree of underlying plaque burden (plaque area) before percutaneous coronary intervention (PCI) and the minimal lumen area achieved after PCI [6]. Prati and colleagues [7] demonstrated with IVUS analysis that late loss (degree of internal hyperplasia) has a direct correlation with the amount of residual plaque burden after stent implantation, which suggests that debulking before stenting might reduce restenosis. Approaching complex lesions is challenging, and lesion preparation with plaque modification (debulking) techniques is suggested as an important adjunct to stenting, which maintains optimal integrity of

the DES delivery platform and polymer by allowing uniform and optimal stent expansion. Routine use of IVUS in addition to good angiographic visualization is suggested in selecting the appropriate plaque modification strategy. Unlike balloon angioplasty or stenting, which widens the coronary lumen merely by displacing atherosclerotic plaque, atherectomy or atherotomy techniques widen the lumen by actually removing tissue from the vessel wall or scoring the plaque in a controlled manner. These plaque modification techniques can be classified into following groups: (1) atherectomy, which removes the plaque using either directional coronary atherectomy (DCA) (Guidant Corp., Indianapolis, Indiana) or rotational atherectomy (RA) (Boston Scientific Corp., Natick, Massachusetts); (2) atherotomy, which cuts (scores) the plaque using low pressure injury using either cutting balloon (CB) (Boston Scientific Corp.) or the FX miniRAIL Balloon (Guidant Corp.); (3) laser angioplasty using excimer laser ablation (Spectranetics Corp., Colorado Springs, Colorado); (4) other innovative newer debulking devices.

Directional coronary atherectomy

The technique of DCA (ie, removing obstructive tissue by a catheter-based excision technique using a nose cone, a metal cutter and housing, and balloon inflation) was approved by the US Food and Drug Administration in 1990. DCA is effective in removing fibrotic, noncalcified plaque, particularly in aorto-ostial, branch ostial, bifurcation, and bulky eccentric lesions in proximal large vessels (size ≥3 mm). Stand-alone DCA has been shown to yield better acute and long-term angiographic results than plain balloon

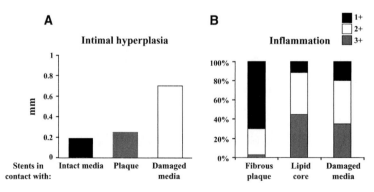

Fig. 1. (*A*) Degree of intimal hyperplasia in relation to vessel wall contact with struts. (*B*) Degree of inflammation related to stent struts contacts.

angioplasty when optimally performed; however, late restenosis still remains high because DCA does not eliminate arterial remodeling and chronic recoil. Coronary stents reduce angiographic restenosis by inhibiting acute recoil and chronic arterial remodeling. The combined approach of debulking followed by stenting has been suggested to overcome the limitations of each device and improve clinical outcomes. Data from several registries suggested the feasibility, safety, and efficacy of performing DCA before stenting, demonstrating low restenosis rates and acceptable acute results in these complex coronary lesions [8]. The encouraging results seen in these registries led to two large, prospective, randomized clinical trials that compared DCA before stenting with stenting alone: the Atherectomy Before MULTI-LINK Improves Lumen Gain and Clinical Outcomes (AMIGO) trial and the Debulking and Stenting In Restenosis Elimination (DESIRE) trial. Long-term (8-month follow-up) results in the AMIGO trial that randomized 753 patients to either DCA followed by stenting or stenting alone showed no difference in angiographic or clinical restenosis between the two groups, with a trend toward lower restenosis rates after optimal debulking. The cumulative major adverse cardiac events (MACE) at 30 days after procedure was slightly higher in the DCA-treated patients [9]. The DESIRE trial randomized 500 patients to

IVUS-guided DCA followed by stenting or stenting alone. Despite the achievement of a lower loss index at follow-up in the DCA + stent group (0.34 versus 0.41 mm), this trial also failed to show a clinical benefit at 6-month follow-up in this group.

Based on the available data, DCA currently is used sparingly in noncalcified ostial left anterior descending and large bifurcation lesions to provide acceptable acute results by reducing plaque shift and improving late angiographic outcome in conjunction with stenting (Fig. 2). The use of DCA has been limited for various reasons, including poor tracking in sharply angulated lesions, difficult feasibility for calcified lesions, long procedure time, risks of perforation, and Dotter effects of the bulky device.

Rotational atherectomy

High-speed RA has been used preferentially in the treatment of heavily calcified, ostial, and undilatable coronary artery lesions. Such lesions are usually associated with lower success and higher complication rates with conventional stenting because of difficulties in stent delivery and expansion. High-pressure, noncompliant balloon inflation for predilatation occasionally may succeed but is often insufficient to overcome vessel wall/plaque resistance and may result in acute recoil, arterial dissections, and perforation. The

DCA & Stent of Ostial LAD Lesion

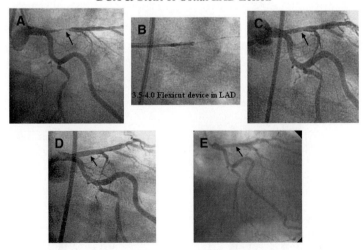

Fig. 2. DCA and stent of ostial left anterior descending coronary artery lesion. (*A*) Angiogram before intervention shows severe stenosis: 90%–95% obstruction of ostial left anterior descending. (*B*) 3.5–4.0 mm Flexicut device in left anterior descending coronary artery. (*C*) An angiogram after 15 cuts at 40 psi. (*D*) The final angiogram shows good results after 3.5/18 mm Cypher stent at 12 atm, with residual obstruction of <10% and no dissections. (*E*) Interventional site with no restenosis (residual <30%) on follow-up angiography 3 years later performed for left circumflex lesion.

technique of RA involves plaque ablation and pulverization by an abrasive diamond coated bur that rotates at approximately 150,000 to 160,000 rpm. Rotablation causes differential cutting, with selective ablation of diseased, inelastic calcified stenosis and produces excellent acute procedural results with relatively low complication rates. The abraded plaque is pulverized into microparticles 5 to 10 μm in diameter that pass through the coronary microcirculation and ultimately undergo phagocytosis in the liver, spleen, and lung. Despite the high acute procedural success rates, RA is plagued by restenosis when used as a stand-alone treatment, perhaps because of chronic arterial recoil and adverse remodeling. It has been reported that successful RA of severely calcified or nondilatable coronary lesions facilitates stent delivery and expansion and reduces plaque shift, which decreases side-branch closure [10,11].

Several nonrandomized, retrospective studies showed improved procedural success rates and a trend toward lower restenosis in calcified lesions with use of RA before stenting versus stenting alone [12–14]. These findings led to two randomized trials that examined the effect of debulking with RA before stenting versus stenting alone. In the Effects of Debulking on Restenosis (EDRES) trial, 150 patients were randomized to stenting alone versus RA with stenting. Although acute gain was identical in both arms, there was reduction in 6-month binary angiographic restenosis in the RA + stenting arm [15]. In the larger Stent Implantation Post Rotational Atherectomy

(SPORT) trial (Fig. 3), 750 patients were randomized to receive either PTCA or RA before stenting. The procedural success rate was better in the RA group; however, there were no differences in angiographic or clinical endpoints between the two groups at 6 to 8 months follow-up [16]. These results may be explained by selection bias in excluding severely calcified lesions to be randomized in the trial. A prospective, randomized trial that compared RA with PTCA before stenting in patients with chronic total occlusion reported that the strategy of debulking before stenting yielded significantly lower angiographic restenosis rates at follow-up [17].

Another set of lesions in which RA has proved beneficial is bifurcation lesions. A major issue with stenting of bifurcation lesions is the snow plough effect and plaque shift into the side branch, which causes severe narrowing or occlusion of the side branch, especially where there is pre-existing ostial disease. Rotablation allows definitive controlled debulking of bulky, sharply angulated calcific bifurcation lesions along with the creation of a channel/gutter to allow the subsequent safe passage of balloons or stents and reduce side-branch closure [18,19].

In summary, RA is recommended before stenting in patients with severely calcified lesions, undilatable lesions, chronic total occlusions, and bifurcation lesions (Fig. 4). Use of this treatment modality requires a high level of training and experience, however, to achieve good results consistently with low rates of complications.

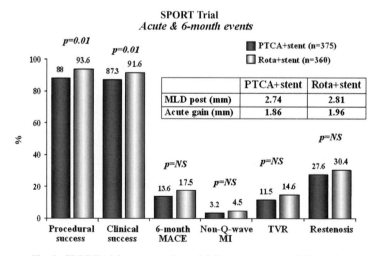

Fig. 3. SPORT trial: acute results and follow-up events at 6–8 months.

Rota+CB of LAD / D1, D2 Bifurcation Calcified Lesion

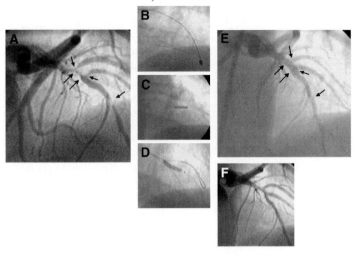

Fig. 4. RA and CB of left anterior descending /D1/D2 bifurcation calcified lesions. (*A*) Right anterior oblique cranial projection before intervention shows severe stenosis: 80%–90% obstruction of mid- left anterior descending, 95% obstruction of distal left anterior descending, 80%–90% D1, and 70%–80% D2. (*B*) A 1.75-mm and then 2.15-mm Rotablator bur is passed through left anterior descending stenosis. (*C*) FXminiRAIL 2.5/10 mm atherotomy in D1. (*D*) CB 2.5/10 mm atherotomy in D2. (*E*) Final angiogram shows good results, with 10% residual obstruction after debulking, dilatation, and stenting (3.5/18 mm Cypher stent) left anterior descending, 10%–30% obstruction of ostial D1, and <10% obstruction of D2. (*F*) Follow-up angiography at 6 months reveals patent PCI sites in left anterior descending /D1/D2.

Cutting balloon angioplasty

The CB device uses three to four longitudinally mounted microsurgical atherotomes on the surface of a noncompliant balloon. The device allows precise scoring of atheromatous plaque and severing continuity of the elastic and fibrotic components of the vessel wall, achieving lumen gain mainly by plaque compression than by vessel wall expansion (Fig. 5 PLUS) [20]. Optimal dilatation

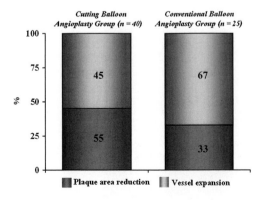

Fig. 5. Mechanisms of lumen enlargement with CB angioplasty versus conventional balloon angioplasty.

of the target lesion is achieved at low-pressure inflations, which potentially minimizes intimal injury and subsequent neointimal proliferation. Although randomized, clinical trials that compared the CB with conventional PTCA showed no differences in acute or long-term clinical and angiographic outcomes, its novel mechanism of action makes CB an attractive tool for lesion preparation before stenting with DES in lesions with high elastic recoil (ostial, bifurcation, or undilatable mildly calcified lesions) [21]. In the Restenosis Reduction by Cutting Balloon Evaluation III (REDUCE III) trial, 521 patients were randomized to CB before ICS (260 patients) or PTCA before stenting (261 patients) with IVUS versus angiographic guidance. At 6-month follow-up, a significantly lower rate of angiographic restenosis was seen with the CB-before-stenting group, mainly in the IVUS-guided group [22].

Use of CB is recommended in ostial, bifurcation, or undilatable mildly calcified lesions before stenting. As a caveat, use of CB PTCA is associated with slightly higher incidence of perforation compared with PTCA. Deliverability also may be an issue with CB PTCA in sharply angulated and tortuous lesions.

FXminiRAIL balloon angioplasty

The FXminiRAIL PTCA catheter (Fig. 6) is an innovative novel approach of lesion modification that applies longitudinal force–focused balloon angioplasty. The catheter consists of an integrated wire outside a semi-compliant dilating balloon and a short monorail with the guidewire lumen located distal to the balloon. This unique dual wire design allows balloon inflation against the standard coronary guidewire and the integrated external wire, which provides concentrated longitudinal scoring of atheromatous plaque along the two wires and creates an expansion plane at low inflation pressures, which facilitates dilatation of resistant and elastic lesions. The safety and efficacy of stand-alone FXminiRAIL PTCA, including its use in mild-to-moderate calcified lesions, have been reported. The efficacy of this technique of plaque modification before stenting is being evaluated in the PreFX Registry, and the preliminary results show a trend toward somewhat better stent expansion after the FXmini-RAIL PTCA [23].

FXminiRAIL PTCA atherotomy may be indicated in ostial and undilatable chronic lesions before stenting. By virtue of its design, FXmini-RAIL is more flexible and deliverable than the CB and can be advanced easily into angulated and less accessible lesions.

Excimer laser coronary angioplasty

First applications of laser technology to the cardiovascular system were in the 1980s. Excimer laser has been used before stenting for aorto-ostial and vein graft lesion with high procedural success (>90%) but no reduction in restenosis and high procedural device and equipment cost. Currently, excimer laser coronary angioplasty has a limited use in lesion modification before stenting.

Other innovative plaque modification devices

Other innovative plaque excision devices, such as the SilverHawk System (Fox Hollow Technologies, Inc., Redwood City, California), AngioSculpt scoring balloon (Angioscore, Inc., Alameda,

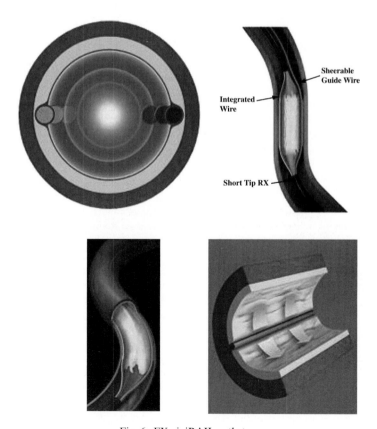

Fig. 6. FXminiRAIL catheter.

California), orbital atherectomy (Cardiovascular Systems, Inc., Santa Clara, California), and Cardio-Path (Pathway Medical Technologies, Inc., Redmond, Washington), are being studied in complex lesions with favorable outcomes. Final results of these trials are awaited before any definite conclusion can be drawn about their effectiveness.

Thrombectomy devices

In recent years research has demonstrated that restoration of normal coronary flow in the infarct-related artery is not necessarily equivalent to the restoration of normal myocardial perfusion through the coronary microcirculation. After conventional primary PCI for ST elevation myocardial infarction (MI) with stent implantation and IIb/IIIa blockade, the normal myocardial perfusion expressed on angiography by the tissue myocardial perfusion grade three is seen in only one third of patients. In the other two thirds of cases, impaired microcirculatory perfusion is observed (tissue myocardial perfusion grade 2-0), accompanied by only partial (30%–70%) or no resolution (<30%) of ST segment elevation in electrocardiography.

Complete resolution of ST segment elevation (>70%) in resting electrocardiography is recognized as a good indicator of restoration of normal myocardial perfusion. Accordingly, patients with impaired microcirculation have increased early and late mortality, greater irreversible myocardial injury, and, consequently, higher incidence of adverse remodeling of the left ventricle, with higher rates of mortality, congestive heart failure, and arrhythmia. One of the main causes of inadequate myocardial reperfusion despite restoration of epicardial flow in the infarct-related artery is embolization of distal artery, side branches, or microcirculation by embolic material that consists of fragmented thrombus, platelet/platelet–leukocyte aggregates, and fragmented plaque released in the course of fibrinolytic therapy or primary PCI. Other reasons include increased microcirculatory resistance caused by neutrophil obstruction, arteriolar constriction, capillary necrosis, progressive myocardial damage, and edema after prolonged ischemia or as a result of reperfusion injury. In extreme cases these phenomena may lead to abrogation of normal rates of epicardial flow despite removal of mechanical obstruction in the infarct-related artery (no reflow) and subsequent attended described adverse sequelae. Thrombus removal may

ameliorate the rate of these adverse sequelae (Fig. 7). Use of glycoprotein (GP) IIb/IIIa inhibitor before PCI has also shown to reduce thrombus burden and subsequent complications [24].

Currently, there are several systems for percutaneous intracoronary thrombectomy. The most widely studied systems are the AngioJet (Possis Medical, Minneapolis, Minnesota) and X-Sizer (eV3) devices. The transluminal extraction catheter is no longer used. Recently, several newer intracoronary thrombectomy devices have been introduced, such as the Export/Transport Catheter (Medtronic, Minneapolis, Minnesota), Diver CE (Invatec Inc., eV3, Plymouth, Minnesota), Pronto (Vascular Solutions, Inc., Minneapolis, Minnesota), Reinspiration (Kerberos Proximal Solutions Inc., Cupertino, California), and simple standard guiding catheters. All these systems differ considerably in construction and principles of operation.

Several small studies have shown improved outcomes in patients who have acute myocardial infarction (AMI) and large thrombus burdens treated with thrombectomy during primary PCI. These initial results in small patient populations were encouraging but so far have not been confirmed in large randomized studies.

Rheolytic thrombectomy with the AngioJet (Possis Medical) is an effective method for removing thrombus by applying the Venturi-Bernoulli vacuum principle. The device (Fig. 8) is a 5-F double lumen, highly flexible catheter that uses a 0.014-in guidewire. Six high-speed saline jets create a low-pressure region at the tip (approximately −760 mm Hg), which acts to pull thrombus and extract it from the vessel. In approaching a lesion with a thrombotic filling defect, the AngioJet device is advanced proximal to

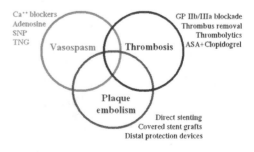

Fig. 7. Coronary intervention of thrombotic lesions: pathophysiology of no-reflow and treatments.

AngioJet Thrombectomy Catheter

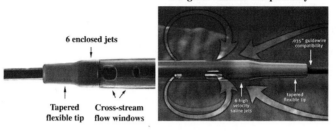

· 6 F guide catheter compatibility

6 enclosed jets

Tapered   Cross-stream
flexible tip   flow windows

Fig. 8. AngioJet thrombectomy catheter.

the lesion and then activated and slowly advanced at approximately 0.5 to 1 mm per second. Repeat passes are performed with angiography after each pass until there is no further improvement in the angiographic appearance of the thrombotic lesion (three to five passes on average). Stent implantation can be performed safely when most of the thrombus has been removed. The device has proved effective in thrombus-containing lesions in the peripheral and coronary circulation and received US Food and Drug Administration approval after showing superiority to urokinase infusion in the VEGAS II Trial [25].

Small studies using AngioJet in AMI have been encouraging. A recently completed multi-center randomized trial of AngioJet Rheolytic Thrombectomy in Patients Undergoing Primary Angioplasty for Acute Myocardial Infarction (AIMI) failed to show any benefit of AngioJet compared with conventional treatment (Fig. 9) [26]. This failure has put the prospects of AngioJet in the treatment of patients who have AMI in severe doubt; however, the serious limitations of the

study have to be recognized, most importantly, absent or minimal thrombus reported in approximately 25% of patients. Baseline TIMI flow-3 was statistically more frequently observed in the control group (27% compared with 19%; $P < 0.05$). Taking this into consideration, it seems that further studies are necessary to finally elucidate the use of Angiojet during primary PCI for AMI with large thrombus burden.

We analyzed our outcomes with or without the AngioJet thrombectomy catheter during primary PCI in patients who have AMI with high-grade thrombus ($\geq$ grade 3, as per TIMI classification) (Box 1) [27]. Ninety-five consecutive patients who had AMI and large thrombotic burden who underwent primary stenting with AngioJet ($n = 52$) and without AngioJet ($n = 43$) were analyzed for the epicardial and microvascular flow and correlated with 30-day MACE and 1-year

Current Standards & Directions for Primary PCI

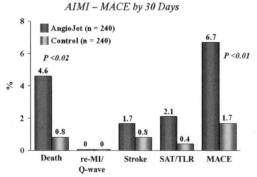

AIMI – MACE by 30 Days

Fig. 9. AngioJet catheter thrombectomy in patients undergoing primary angioplasty for AMI.

Box 1. Thrombus grades: TIMI thrombus grade

- Grade 0: No thrombus
- Grade 1: Possible thrombus (mural opacities)
- Grade 2: Small thrombus (<0.5λ normal lumen diameter)
- Grade 3: Medium thrombus (0.5–1.5λ normal lumen diameter)
- Grade 4: Large thrombus (>1.5λ normal lumen diameter)
- Grade 5: Recent thrombotic occlusion (fresh thrombus with dye stasis and delayed washout)
- Grade 6: Chronic total occlusion (smooth, abrupt, and with no dye stasis and brisk flow)

survival. Results showed that use of the AngioJet thrombectomy catheter during primary stenting of patients who have AMI with high-grade thrombus resulted in better epicardial and microvascular flow, which resulted in improved short- and long-term outcomes (Table 1). Our findings are in contrast with the lack of benefit of AngioJet use in the AIMI trial, perhaps because of the different exclusion criteria (in the AIMI trial, all patients were included, regardless of the thrombus grade, whereas our trial included only patients with high-grade thrombus).

It has been demonstrated that thrombectomy with X-Sizer (Fig. 10) before stent implantation during primary PCI for AMI effectively decreases thrombus mass in the culprit lesion, which allows restoration of TIMI- 3 flow in a large proportion of patients and prevents slow-flow, no-reflow, and distal embolization, as measured by improved myocardial perfusion by angiography and improved ST segment elevation resolution at 60 minutes after PCI. The system's helix cutter is housed within an atraumatic catheter tip. Fully assembled and completely disposable, the X-Sizer catheter system can be set up, used, and disposed of in a matter of minutes (Fig. 11). The X-Sizer catheter combines vacuum technology with a patented helix cutter housed in the tip of a small catheter. When engaged, the system creates a powerful vacuum effect designed to capture and remove occlusive material. The Archimedes screw is designed to grab thrombus on contact and quickly draw it in, shearing and removing it. A randomized trial, the X-Tract trial, which compared X-sizer and conventional treatment, failed to show any difference in 30-day MACE but did show reduced large MI (Table 2).

Technical limitations of X-Sizer must be acknowledged. The significant rigidity of the

Table 1
AngioJet thrombectomy catheter during primary stenting of patients with high-grade thrombus

	AngioJet ($n = 52$)	Non-AngioJet ($n = 43$)	P
Age (y)	62 ± 14	66 ± 15	NS
Anterior MI (%)	65	70	NS
Pain-to-door time (hr)	14 ± 3	12 ± 4	NS
Door-to-balloon time (min)	183 ± 32	169 ± 62	NS
LVEF (%)	44 ± 10	42 ± 10	NS
TIMI before PCI (%)	0.66 ± 0.98	0.93 ± 1.14	0.24
Thrombus grade (%)	4.6	4.3	NS
TIMI after PCI (%)	2.7	2.2	0.007
TMP grade (mean)	2.16 ± 10	1.53 ± 1.1	0.006
TMP grade 2/3 (%)	66	43	0.01
CTFC (mean)	22 ± 13	28 ± 11	0.02
30-day MACE (%)	6	11	0.12
1-year mortality (%)	7.4	14.6	0.08
Event-free survival at 1 year (%)	86	74	0.05

Abbreviations: CTFC, corrected TIMI frame count; LVEF, left ventricle ejection fraction; TMP, TIMI myocardial perfusion; TIMI, thrombolysis in myocardial infarction.

catheter decreases its ability to cope with tortuosity and excessive calcification proximal to the culprit lesion. Its large profile prevents crossing of tight lesions and limits its use with arteries with reference diameter > 2.5 mm. The presence of the cutting blade in conjunction with difficult anatomy increases the risk of vessel perforation.

Numerous old and emerging thrombectomy devices work mainly on the principle of aspiration: Transluminal Extraction Catheter (Interventional Therapeutics, Minneapolis, Minnesota), Rescue (Boston Scientific Corp.), Export/Transport Catheter (Medtronic), Pronto Extraction

Angiojet Thrombectomy for Thrombotic LCx Lesion in AMI

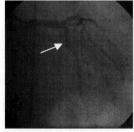 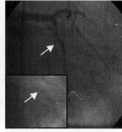 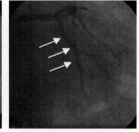

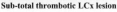

| Sub-total thrombotic LCx lesion | Post AngioJet thrombectomy | 0–10% residual post 4.0/23.0 mm Zeta stent, with final TIMI III flow and TMP grade III |

Fig. 10. AngioJet thrombectomy for thrombotic LCx lesion in AMI. LCx, left circumflex.

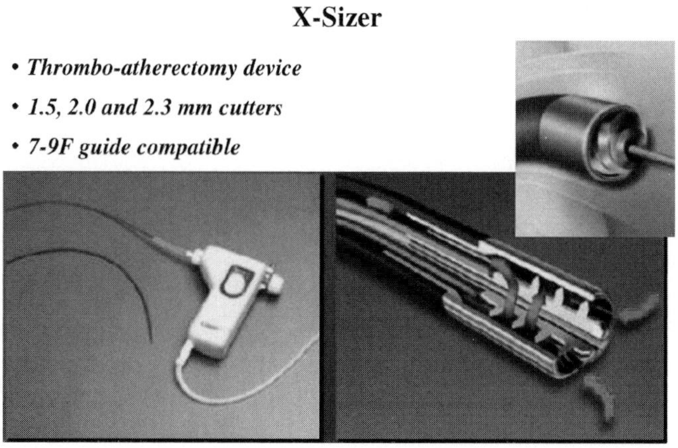

X-Sizer

- *Thrombo-atherectomy device*
- *1.5, 2.0 and 2.3 mm cutters*
- *7-9F guide compatible*

Fig. 11. The X-Sizer catheter.

Catheter (Vascular Solutions, Inc.), Diver CE (Invatec Inc.), and Reinspiration (Kerberos Proximal Solutions Inc.). Trials involving these aspiration catheters are small, with variable success, but they may play a role in the catheterization laboratory because of ease of use and deliverability, reduced bulkiness, and fast setup (Tables 2 and 3).

Distal protection devices

Percutaneous intervention of diseased saphenous vein grafts (SVGs) is known to be associated with a high periprocedural rate of complications [28]. Distal protection systems are based on either occlusive distal balloons (PercuSurge GuardWire) or filter-based devices. Two distal protection devices (GuardWire and Filter WireEX) have proved to be clinically beneficial for PCI of SVG lesions. The hope that distal protection may improve results of PCI of thrombotic lesions is based on the fact that these systems provide protection from distal embolization during each balloon inflation and stent implantation, while thrombectomy is performed only before stent implantation. Distal protection during SVG PCI using a balloon occlusion and aspiration system (the PercuSurge GuardWire) has been shown in a large randomized trial to reduce 30-day MACE rates by 42% (Saphenous vein graft Angioplasty Free of Emboli Randomized, SAFER Trial) (Table 2) [29]. Compared with balloon occlusion systems, filter-based distal protection devices may be simpler to use and allow antegrade perfusion during the procedure, which reduces ischemia time and facilitates intervention in patients with poor left ventricular

function. The absolute clinical efficacy of distal filters as an adjunct to PCI for diseased SVGs has not been proven (Fig. 12). The relative efficacy of two distal protection devices was compared in a randomized trial (see Table 2). The FIRE trial was a large, multicenter trial of PCI in diseased SVGs in which 650 consecutive patients at 65 US and Canadian centers were randomized 1:1 to intervention with distal protection using the BSC/EPI FilterWire EX versus the PercuSurge GuardWire. The FilterWire consists of a microporous polyurethane net attached to a self-expanding nitinol ring anchored distally to a 0.014-in guidewire over which PCI is performed. Randomization was stratified by use of IIb/IIIa inhibitors. The primary endpoint was the composite rate of death, mL (CPK-MB 3× normal values), coronary artery bypass graft, or target lesion revascularization at 30 days. The mean graft age was 11 ± 8 years. The trial showed equal efficacy of both distal protection devices [30].

Promising results with PercuSurge GuardWire or Filterwire in SVG have not yet been confirmed in the larger randomized studies of AMI, such as the Enhanced Myocardial Efficacy and Removal by Aspiration of Liberated Debris (EMERALD) study. Despite the fact that thrombotic and plaque debris were found in aspirates of 76% of patients, no differences were found between studied groups in angiographically assessed myocardial reperfusion, ST segment elevation resolution, or infarct size measured by isotope scan at 30 days. The results of the EMERALD trial have impeached seriously the concept of mechanical cardioprotection of the microcirculation during primary PCI for AMI [31]. The PercuSurge

Table 2
Completed trails using embolic protection in coronary intervention

Trial name	Clinical syndrome	Device	No. patients	Management strategy	Other agents used	Endpoint	Results (intervention vs. control)
SAFE	Elective SVG intervention (low thrombus burden)	GuardWire	105	Registry		In-hospital MACE final TIMI grade 3 flow	5% 99%
SAFER	Elective SVG intervention	GuardWire vs. no distal protection	801	Prospective, randomized trial	GP IIb/IIIa inhibitor in approximately 58%	30-day MACE	9.6% 16.5% P = 0.004
FilterWire during SVG stenting	Elective SVG intervention	Filter Wire	60 (phase 1) 248 (phase 2)	Registry	GP IIb/IIIa inhibitor in 30%–50%	30-day MACE	21% (phase 1) 11% (phase 2)
FIRE	Elective SVG intervention (low thrombus burden)	Filter Wire vs. GuardWire	651	Prospective, randomized trial	GP IIb/IIIa inhibitor in approximately 52% lesions	30-day MACE	10% vs. 12%
X-TRACT	SVG (70%) or thrombus-rich native vessel (30%)	X-Sizer vs. no DPD	50 (phase 1) 797 (phase 2)	Prospective, randomized trial	GP IIb/IIIa inhibitor in approximately 76% lesions in both arms	30-day MACE, Large AMI (CKMB >8X ULN)	17% vs. 17%, P = NS 5% vs. 10%, P = 0.002
PRIDE	SVG	TriActive vs. Filter Wire/GuardWire	631	Prospective, randomized trial	GP IIb IIIa inhibitor in approximately 54% in both arms	30-day MACE	11% vs. 12%, P = NS
CAPTIVE	SVG	Cardio Shield vs. GuardWire	652	Prospective, randomized trial	Uncertain, pending full trial publication	30-day MACE	10% vs. 12%, P = NS

Abbreviations: CKMB, creatine kinase isoenzyme MB; DPD, distales protection device; SVG, saphenous vein graft; ULN, upper limit of normal.

Table 3
Ongoing trials using embolic protection in coronary intervention

Trial name	Clinical syndrome	Device	No. patients	Management strategy	Other agents used	Endpoint	Results (intervention vs. control)
PROXIMAL	SVG intervention	Proximal protection device	Proxis	600	Randomized to Proxis or other DPD	30-day MACE	Completed equal efficacy
DEAR-MI	AMI	Thrombectomy	Pronto	200	Randomized to Pronto thrombectomy vs. no treatment	ST-segment resolution LV function recovery	Ongoing
RULE-SVG	PCI to SVG	Filter	Rubicon	60	Randomized to Rubicon vs. no protection	30-day MACE	Ongoing
SPIDER	PCI to SVG	Filter	SpideRX	770	Randomized to SpideRX or GuardWire	30-day MACE	Ongoing
GUARD	PCI to SVG	Filter	Angioguard	800	Randomized to AngioGuard or GuardWire	30-day MACE	Ongoing
AMEthyst	PCI to SVG	Filter	Interceptor	600	Randomized to Interceptor or GuardWire	30-day MACE	Ongoing

Abbreviation: DPD, distales protection device.

Filterwire in SVG to LCx lesion

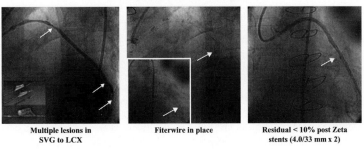

| Multiple lesions in SVG to LCX | Fiterwire in place | Residual < 10% post Zeta stents (4.0/33 mm x 2) |

Fig. 12. Filterwire in SVG to left circumflex (LCx) lesion.

GuardWire system has important limitations. Aspiration of thromboembolic material is performed via an ordinary perfusion catheter without the thrombus fragmentation, which is in contradiction to the AngioJet or X-Sizer. This approach may result in the inability to remove large fragments of thrombotic debris. The GuardWire balloon is inflated 3 to 5cm beyond the occlusion site and as such has no ability to prevent distal embolization of side branches that originate in between.

Two new combined embolic protection and thrombectomy devices have been introduced for SVG interventions (see Tables 2 and 3). The Proxis-device (Velocimed, Minneapolis, Minnesota) consists of a short, flexible catheter (internal diameter, 0.058 in) attached to a hypertube-catheter shaft with a short circumferential balloon at the distal tip. The device is introduced through an 8-F guiding catheter and advanced in the proximal part of the occluded artery. The balloon at the tip of the device is inflated at 2 atm; wire crossing of the coronary occlusion, balloon dilatation, and stent placement are performed through the device under total proximal blockade of the vessel. After withdrawal of dilatation or stent balloons, aspiration of debris is performed and continuses when coronary flow is restored by deflation of the device balloon. Temporary proximal vessel occlusion and aspiration are repeated during each step of the PCI procedure. The preliminary results suggest that the device is effective for aspiration of embolic elements.

Another distal protection device based on balloon occlusion and aspiration, the TriActive System, was evaluated in the Protection During Saphenous Vein Graft Intervention to Prevent Distal Embolization (PRIDE) study against other distal protection devices. The PRIDE study compared outcomes with the TriActive System

(Kensey Nash Corp., Exton, Pennsylvania), a balloon-protection flush and extraction device, with an embolic protection group during treatment of SVGs. The incidence of major adverse cardiac events at 30 days was 11.2% for the TriActive group and 10.1% for the control group ($P = 0.65$; $P = 0.02$ for noninferiority). Slightly higher vascular complications were reported in the TriActive group [32].

Summary

Percutaneous treatment of thrombus-containing lesions is associated with higher complication rates compared with nonthrombotic lesions. Adjunct devices, such as thrombectomy or distal protection, are commonly used as part of the interventional procedure along with the liberal use of GP IIb/IIIa inhibitors or vasodilators (Fig. 13). Percutaneous treatment of SVG using distal protection (PercuSurge or filter devices) is routinely recommended with stent implantation to improve short- and long-term results. Despite achieving TIMI-3 flow, myocardial perfusion in AMI

Treatment Options for Thrombotic Lesions (SVG or native)

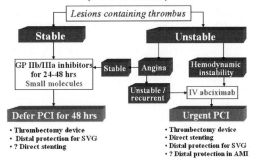

Fig. 13. Treatment options for thrombotic lesions (SVG or native).

remains suboptimal in a significant number of patients, resulting in larger final infarct size. Effective removal of thrombi before stenting theoretically may reduce distal embolization of thrombus, which could improve myocardial perfusion and salvage. Randomized studies do not support routine use of thrombectomy devices or distal protection devices with primary PCI in all patients who have AMI for the reduction of major adverse cardiac events. Simple manual aspiration with easy-to-use catheters to extract atherothrombotic material from target lesions, which restores flow and increases patency rate of an infarct-related artery before stenting, may be the hypothetical option for selected patients during primary PCI.

References

[1] Moses JW, Leon MB, Popma JJ, et al. Sirolimus-eluting stents versus standard stents in patients with stenosis in a native coronary artery. N Engl J Med 2003;349:1315–23.

[2] Stone GW, Ellis SG, Cox D, et al. A polymerbased, paclitaxel-eluting stent in patients with coronary artery disease. N Engl J Med 2004;350:221–31.

[3] Fujii K, Mintz GS, Kobayashi Y, et al. Contribution of stent underexpansion to recurrence after sirolimus-eluting stent implantation for in-stent restenosis. Circulation 2004;109:1085–8.

[4] Takebayashi H, Mintz G, Carlier S, et al. Nonuniform strut distribution correlates with more neointimal hyperplasia after sirolimus-eluting stent implantation. Circulation 2004;110:3430–4.

[5] Farb A, Sangiorgi G, Carter A, et al. Pathology of acute and chronic coronary stenting in humans. Circulation 1999;99:44–52.

[6] Takeda Y, Tsuchikane E, Kobayashi T, et al. Effect of plaque debulking before stent implantation on in-stent neointimal proliferation: a serial 3-dimensional intravascular ultrasound study. Am Heart J 2003; 146:175–82.

[7] Prati F, Mario C, Moussa I, et al. In-stent neointimal proliferation correlates with the amount of residual plaque burden outside the stent: an intravascular ultrasound study. Circulation 1999; 99:1011–4.

[8] Moussa I, Moses J, Di Mario C, et al. Stenting after optimal lesion debulking (SOLD) registry: angiographic and clinical outcome. Circulation 1998;98: 1604–9.

[9] Stankovic G, Colombo A, Bersin R, et al. Comparison of directional coronary atherectomy and stenting versus stenting alone for the treatment of de novo and restenotic coronary artery narrowing. Am J Cardiol 2004;93:953–8.

[10] Reifart N, Vandormael M, Krajcar M, et al. Randomized comparison of angioplasty of complex coronary lesions at a single center: excimer laser, rotational atherectomy, and balloon angioplasty comparison (ERBAC) study. Circulation 1997;96: 91–8.

[11] Kini A, Marmur J, Duvvuri S, et al. Rotational atherectomy: improved procedural outcome with evolution of technique and equipment. Single-center results of first 1,000 patients. Catheter Cardiovasc Interv 1999;46:305–11.

[12] Chung CM, Nakamura S, Tanaka K, et al. Stenting alone versus debulking and debulking plus stent in branch ostial lesions of native coronary arteries. Heart Vessels 2004;19:213–20.

[13] Cavusoglu E, Kini A, Marmur J, et al. Current status of rotational atherectomy. Catheter Cardiovasc Interv 2004;62:485–98.

[14] Kini A, Kim M, Das S, et al. Efficacy of drug-eluting stents in calcified lesions. J Am Coll Cardiol 2005; 45(Suppl A):65A.

[15] Dunn B. The effects of debulking on restenosis (EDRES). J Saudi Heart Assn 1998;10:55.

[16] Buchbinder M, Fortuna R, Sharma S, et al. Debulking prior to stenting improves acute outcomes: early results from the SPORT trial. J Am Coll Cardiol 2000;35(Suppl A):8A.

[17] Tsuchikane E, Suzuki T, Asakura Y, et al. Debulking of chronic total occlusions with rotational or directional atherectomy before stenting trial: a multicenter randomized study [abstract]. J Am Coll Cardiol 2004;43:59A.

[18] Sharma SK. Simultaneous kissing drug-eluting stent technique for percutaneous treatment of bifurcation lesions in large-size vessels. Catheter Cardiovasc Interv 2005;65:10–6.

[19] Tan R, Kini A, Shalouh E, et al. Optimal treatment of nonaorto ostial coronary lesions in large vessels: acute and long-term results. Catheter Cardiovasc Interv 2001;54:283–8.

[20] Hara H, Nakamura M, Asahara T, et al. Intravascular ultrasonic comparison of mechanisms of vasodilatation of cutting balloon angioplasty versus conventional balloon angioplasty. Am J Cardiol 2002;89:1253–6.

[21] Mauri L, Bonan R, Weiner BH, et al. Cutting balloon angioplasty for the prevention of restenosis: results of the cutting balloon global randomized trial. Am J Cardiol 2002;90:1079–83.

[22] Ozaki Y, Suzuki T, Yamaguchi T, et al. Can intravascular ultrasound guided cutting balloon angioplasty before stenting be a substitute for drug eluting stent? Final results of the prospective randomized multicenter trial comparing cutting balloon with balloon angioplasty before stenting (Reduce III) [abstract]. J Am Coll Cardiol 2004; 43:82A.

[23] Ischinger TA, Solar RJ, Hitzke E. Improved outcome with novel device for low-pressure PTCA in de novo and in-stent lesions. Cardiovasc Radiat Med 2003;4:2–6.

[24] Zhao XQ, Théroux P, Snapinn SM, et al. Intracoronary thrombus and platelet glycoprotein IIb/IIIa receptor blockade with tirofiban in unstable angina or non–Q-wave myocardial infarction: angiographic results from the PRISM-PLUS trial (platelet receptor inhibition for ischemic syndrome management in patients limited by unstable signs and symptoms). Circulation 1999;100:1609–15.

[25] Kuntz R, Baim D, Cohen D, et al. A trial comparing rheolytic thrombectomy with intracoronary urokinase for coronary and vein graft thrombus (the Vein Graft AngioJet Study [VeGAS 2]). Am J Cardiol 2002;89:326–30.

[26] Ali A, on behalf of the AIMI Investigators. AngioJet rheolytic thrombectomy in patients undergoing primary angioplasty for acute myocardial infarction. Presented at the Transcatheter Cardiovascular Therapeutics conference. Washington, DC, September 2004.

[27] Tamburrino F, Kini A, Gupta S, et al. The improved outcome with AngioJet thrombectomy catheter during primary stenting in acute myocardial infarction patients with high-grade thrombus. Am J Cardiol 2005;96(Suppl 7A):76H.

[28] Hong MK, Mehran R, Dangas G, et al. Creatine kinase-MB enzyme elevation following successful saphenous vein graft intervention is associated with late mortality. Circulation 1999;100:2400–5.

[29] Baim DS, Wahr D, George B, et al. Randomized trial of a distal embolic protection device during percutaneous intervention of saphenous vein aorto-coronary bypass grafts. Circulation 2002;105:1285–90.

[30] Stone G, Rogers C, Hermiller J, et al. Randomized comparison of distal protection with a filter-based catheter and a balloon occlusion and aspiration system during percutaneous intervention of diseased saphenous vein aorto-coronary bypass grafts. Circulation 2003;108:548–53.

[31] Stone GW, Webb J, Cox DA, et al. Distal microcirculatory protection during percutaneous coronary intervention in acute ST-segment elevation myocardial infarction: a randomized controlled trial. JAMA 2005;293:1063–72.

[32] Carrozza J, Mumma M, Breall J, et al. Randomized evaluation if the TriActiv balloon-protection flush and extraction system for the treatment of saphenous vein graft disease. J Am Coll Cardiol 2005;46: 1677–83.

ELSEVIER
SAUNDERS

Cardiol Clin 24 (2006) 217–231

CARDIOLOGY
CLINICS

Drug-Eluting Stents

Jeffrey J. Popma, MD*, Mark Tulli, MD

*Department of Internal Medicine (Cardiovascular Division), Brigham and Women's Hospital,
75 Francis Street, Boston, MA 02115, USA*

Percutaneous coronary intervention (PCI) has evolved dramatically over the past 25 years. Stand-alone balloon angioplasty has been replaced with the use of coronary stents because of the near elimination of emergency coronary artery bypass surgery (CABG) [1] and marked reductions in restenosis associated with the use of coronary stents [2,3]. With the introduction of dozens of balloon-expandable stents during the mid- and late 1990s, progressive improvements in the crossing profile, deliverability, and metallic composition occurred, albeit with little change in the overall occurrence of stent restenosis [4–6]. Clinical restenosis associated with stent use was particularly frequent (up to 30%) in patients who had small vessels, long lesions, and diabetes mellitus [7].

A breakthrough occurred in early 2000 with the development of stents that eluted pharmacology agents directly into the vessel wall by means of a controlled release from a durable polymer coating. Various drug-eluting stents (DES) were developed, each varying with its delivery platform, polymer coating (or absence of coating), and drug selected for elution. This article describes the clinically available and late developmental drug-eluting stent programs targeted for treating patients who have coronary artery disease.

Sirolimus-eluting stents

The CYPHER stent (Cordis Corporation, Miami Lakes, Florida) is composed of balloon-expandable stainless steel, a durable copolymer mixture of polyethylene–covinyl acetate (PEVA) and poly-n-butyl methacrylate (PBMA), and a sirolimus, which is a G1 cell cycle inhibitor that also has potent anti-inflammatory properties. Using the commercially available, slow-release polymer formulation, 90% of the sirolimus contained on the stent is released within 30 days [8]. The CYPHER stent was approved for clinical use in Europe in April 2002 and in the United States in May 2003. This stent is used in approximately 50% of DES procedures worldwide.

First in man studies

Much has been learned about the late-term (4-year) safety and efficacy of the CYPHER stent from the first 45 patients with focal native vessel disease who were treated with slow-release (release over 30 days) and fast-release (release over 7 to 10 days) sirolimus-eluting stents (SES) [9–11]. Serial evaluation at 4 months [9], 1 year [12], 2 years [13], and 4 years [11] showed a minimal degree (less than 0.10 mm) of intimal hyperplasia within the stent at each of these follow-up intervals, and no late untoward toxicities, such as acquired late aneurysms. Although the target vessel revascularization (TLR) rate for the entire cohort was 10% at 2 years [13], there were no TLRs or stent thromboses (STs) that developed between 2- and 4-year follow-up [11]. In-stent late lumen loss was slightly greater at 4 years in the fast-release group (0.41 ± 0.49 mm) than in the slow-release group (0.09 ± 0.23 mm). Similarly, intravascular ultrasound showed a slightly higher degree of volume obstruction in the fast-release group (9.1%) compared with the slow-release group (5.7%) [11], suggesting that release kinetics may play an important role in the efficacy of SES.

---

* Corresponding author.
E-mail address: jpopma@partners.org (J.J. Popma).

0733-8651/06/$ - see front matter © 2006 Elsevier Inc. All rights reserved.
doi:10.1016/j.ccl.2006.04.001

cardiology.theclinics.com

RAVEL

The RAVEL trial was a randomized study of 238 patients who had single, focal lesions located in larger native coronary arteries and who were assigned to treatment with SES or a bare metal stent (BMS). It was the first controlled study to show a marked reduction in clinical and angiographic restenosis in patients treated with SES [14]. There were no cases of binary angiographic restenosis in patients treated with SES compared with a 26.6% incidence in patients assigned to treatment with BMS ($P < .001$) [15]. One analysis suggested that early and late side branch patency improved with the use of SES [16]. Volumetric intravascular ultrasound analysis found a 90% reduction in intimal hyperplasia in those treated with SES [17]. Clinical benefits associated with the use of SES were sustained up to 3 years later, with 93.7% of patients assigned to treatment with SES being free from TLR compared with 75.0% in patients assigned to treatment with BMS ($P < .001$) [18]. Three-year major adverse cardiac events (MACE) developed in 15.8% of patients in the SES group and in 33.1% of patients in the BMS group ($P = .002$) [18].

SIRIUS

The SIRIUS trial was a randomized comparison of 1058 patients who had complex coronary artery disease that included lesion lengths between 15 and 30 mm and vessel diameters between 2.5 mm and 3.5 mm and who were assigned to treatment with SES or BMS [8]. The overall complexity of patients enrolled in the study was confirmed by the frequent presence of diabetes mellitus (26%), long lesions (lesion length 14.4 mm), and smaller vessel size (mean diameter 2.80 mm). The primary end point was target vessel failure, defined as a composite of death from cardiac causes, myocardial infarction (MI), or target vessel revascularization within 270 days. These events were reduced from 21.0% in patients assigned to BMS compared with 8.6% in those assigned to SES ($P < .001$). The need for TLR was reduced from 16.6% in those assigned to treatment with BMS compared with 4.1% in those assigned to SES ($P < .001$). These benefits were consistent across all patient and lesion subsets. Although there were no differences in the occurrence of death or MI, at 1-year follow-up, the absolute difference in TLR continued to increase (20% in patients assigned to treatment with

BMS and 4.9% in patients assigned to treatment with SES; $P < .001$) [19].

The clinical benefit in this study was caused by the profound reduction in intimal hyperplasia within the SES compared with a BMS. Angiographic restudy was obtained in 701 patients enrolled in the SIRIUS trial 240 days after stent placement [20]. Patients treated with SES had lower rates of binary (greater than 50% follow-up diameter stenosis) angiographic restenosis within the segment (8.9% versus 36.3% with BMS; $P < .001$) and within the stent (3.2% versus 35.4% with BMS, $P < .001$). SES had less late lumen loss within the treated segment (0.24 ± 0.47 mm versus 0.81 ± 0.67 with BMS, $P < .001$), within the stent (0.17 mm ± 0.44 versus 1.00 ± 0.70 mm, respectively; $P < .001$), and within its 5 mm proximal (0.16 ± 0.48 mm versus 0.32 ± 0.63 mm, respectively; $P < .001$) and distal (0.04 ± 0.24 mm versus 0.24 ± 0.61 mm, respectively; $P < .001$) edges 8 months after stent placement. The frequency of late aneurysms was similar in the two groups.

E-SIRIUS

The European extension to SIRIUS, known as E-SIRIUS, enrolled 352 patients who had single native coronary lesions with a vessel diameter 2.5 to 3.0 mm and lesion length 15 to 32 mm. Patients were assigned randomly to treatment with SES or BMS [21]. Although the frequency of diabetes was less in the E-SIRIUS study than in the SIRIUS study, the mean vessel diameter was slightly smaller (2.55 ± 0.37 mm), and the mean lesion length was longer (15.0 ± 6.0 mm) than in patients enrolled in SIRIUS. Fewer patients assigned to treatment with SES experienced a 9 month major adverse cardiac event (MACE) (8.0% versus 22.6% in patients assigned to BMS, $P = .0002$). This was primarily because of a reduction in the need for TLR (4.0% versus 20.9% in patients assigned to BMS, $P < .0001$). The binary angiographic restenosis rate 8 months later was reduced significantly in the SES group (5.9% versus 42.3% in the BMS group; $P = .0001$). Because of meticulous attention to deployment technique, including the avoidance of balloon inflations at the stent margins, the occurrence of edge restenosis was reduced in the E-SIRIUS study compared with the SIRIUS study.

C-SIRIUS

The Canadian SIRIUS study enrolled 100 patients at eight Canadian sites with similar inclusion criteria to the SIRIUS and E-SIRIUS studies [22]. Angiographic restenosis developed in one (2.3%) patient assigned to treatment with SES and in 23 (52%) patients assigned to treatment with a BMS (52.3%, $P < .001$). Two (4%) patients required TLRs by 270 days in the SES group compared with 18% in patients assigned to treatment with BMS ($P = .05$).

Stent restenosis

Stent restenosis is an increasingly uncommon cause of recurrent ischemia after stent placement, owing to the more frequent use of DES in patients undergoing PCI. Yet when stent restenosis does occur, treatment options include the use of brachytherapy, angioplasty with conventional or cutting balloons, or DES placement [23–25]. Clinical event rates were low in a series of 25 patients with relatively focal stent restenosis who were treated with one or two SES [23], whereas patients with more complex in-stent restenosis had higher events rates, often relating to thrombosis within the stent, despite a minimal degree of intimal hyperplasia within the stent [26].

In the Sirolimus-eluting stent for In-Stent Restenosis (SISR) trial, 384 patients were assigned randomly to treatment with vascular brachytherapy using gamma or beta sources or to placement of one or more SES [27]. Patients were included if the stent restenosis occurred in vessels with a diameter between 2.5 and 3.5 mm, and the stent restenosis was between 15 and 40 mm in length. The primary endpoint, target vessel failure, was reduced from 21.6% in patients assigned to treatment with brachytherapy to 12.4% in patients assigned to treatment with DES ($P = .023$). At the time of follow-up angiography, there was a trend toward improvement in the analysis segment binary angiographic restenosis rate in patients treated with the SES (19.5% versus 29.5% in the brachytherapy treated patients, $P = .067$). There were two late stent thromboses in patients assigned to treatment with SES. These data suggest that long-term dual antiplatelet therapy may be needed to prevent late stent thrombosis.

SIRIUS registries and subset analyses

Acute coronary syndromes

As part of the Rapamycin-Eluting Stent Evaluated At Rotterdam Cardiology Hospital (RESEARCH) registry, 198 patients presenting with an acute coronary syndrome and treated with a SES were compared with a control group of 301 patients with a similar presentation who were treated with BMS [28]. The 30-day major adverse cardiac event rate was similar in both groups (6.1% in SES patients versus 6.6% in control patients, $P = .8$), including the occurrence of stent thrombosis (0.5% in SES patients versus 1.7% in control patients, $P = .4$). Using the same RESEARCH registry, the late clinical outcomes in patients with ST segment myocardial infarction (STEMI) were compared in 186 consecutive patients treated with SES and 183 patients treated with BMS [29]. Stent thrombosis did not occur in any patient treated with the SES but occurred in 1.6% of patients treated with BMS. Those treated with SES had a reduced incidence of combined adverse events at 300 days significantly (9.4% compared with 17% in patients treated with BMS, $P = .02$), primarily because of a lower risk of TLR in patients treated with SES (1.1% compared with 8.2% in patients treated with BMS, $P = .01$) [29]. The data support the use of SES in patients who present with an acute coronary syndrome, including STEMI.

Diabetic patients

In the SIRIUS trial, the 279 patients who had a history of diabetes mellitus were treated with SES or BMS [30]. Late (270 day) TLR was reduced in diabetic patients from 22.3% with BMS to 6.9% with SES ($P < .001$), and late MACE was reduced from 25% with BMS to 9.2% with SES ($P < .001$). Although SES was markedly effective in reducing in stent intimal hyperplasia, edge restenosis often occurred in these diabetic patients, because of either balloon injury not covered with SES or oversizing of the SES in diffusely diseased vessels.

Small coronary arteries

In a multi-center, prospective trial, 257 patients were randomized to treatment with SES or BMS for lesions in native coronary arteries no more than 2.75 mm [31]. The mean vessel diameter was 2.2 ± 0.28 mm, and the lesion length was 11.8 ± 6.2 mm. The primary endpoint, 8-month binary in-segment restenosis rate, occurred in 9.8% of patients in the SES group and in 53.1% patients in the BMS group (risk reduction (RR), 0.18; $P < .001$). Late MACE occurred in 9.3% patients assigned to treatment with SES and in 31.3% patients assigned to treatment with BMS (RR, 0.30; $P < .001$), primary because of reductions in TLR (7% versus 21.1%, respectively; RR, 0.33; $P = .002$) and MI (1.6% versus 7.8%, respectively; RR, 0.20; $P = .04$).

Other patient and lesion subsets

The beneficial effect of SES over BMS has been demonstrated in numerous complex subsets, including patients with chronic total occlusion [32], saphenous vein graft disease [33,34], left main coronary artery disease [35–38], bifurcation lesions [39–41], and diffuse disease requiring four or more stents [42]. Direct stenting with SES is also as effective as SES placement after redilation [43].

Durable polymer, paclitaxel-eluting stents

The TAXUS stent (Boston Scientific, Natick, Massachusetts) is comprised of a stainless steel stent platform, a polyolefin polymer derivative, and a microtubular stabilizing agent paclitaxel, with two-phase 30-day polymeric release kinetics that provide its antiproliferative effect [44]. Paclitaxel is an inhibitor of microtubules that prevents cell division at the M phase. Paclitaxel release is completed within 30 days of implantation, although a substantial portion (greater than 90%) of the paclitaxel remains within the polymer indefinitely.

The TAXUS-I trial

The TAXUS-I Trial was a prospective, randomized study of 61 patients with de novo or restenotic lesions who received a paclitaxel-eluting stent (PES) or BMS [45]. There were no cases of angiographic restenosis 6 months after the procedure in patients treated with PES, compared with a 10% restenosis rate in patients treated with a BMS. The low composite MACE rates reported at 1-year follow-up (3.2% in patients treated with PES compared with 10.0% in patients with BMS) were maintained at 2 and 3 years, with no additional MACE in either treatment group 1 year after implantation [46].

The TAXUS-II trial

TAXUS-II was a large randomized trial in 536 patients with native vessel coronary artery disease who were assigned randomly to treatment with

BMS (NIR Express; Boston Scientific, Natick, Massachusetts) or PES using either a slow (SR)- or moderate release (MR)- polymeric coating [47]. The primary study endpoint, 6-month in-stent net percent volume obstruction measured by intravascular ultrasound, was significantly lower for PES (7.9% SR and 7.8% MR) than for SES (23.2% and 20.5%, $P < .0001$ for both). Angiographic restenosis was reduced from 17.9% in the BMS cohort to 2.3% in the PES-SR cohort ($P < .0001$) and from 20.2% in the BMS cohort to 4.7% in the PES-MR cohort ($P = .0002$). A serial intravascular ultrasound study demonstrated that the marked reduction in in-stent restenosis with SR or MR stents was not associated with increased edge stenosis at 6-month follow-up IVUS [48]. Compared with BMS, there was a reduction in late lumen loss at the distal edge with TAXUS stents [48]. Twelve-month MACE was also lower in the TAXUS-SR (10.9%) and TAXUS-MR (9.9%) groups than in controls (22.0% and 21.4%, respectively), in large part because of a reduction in TLR in patients who were treated with PES [47].

TAXUS-III

Twenty-eight patients who had complex in-stent restenosis were treated with PES (NIR platform) in the TAXUS-III study [49]. Although no subacute stent thromboses occurred within the first 12 months, the MACE rate was 29%, including six patients who required TLR. The high recurrence rate was attributable to the development of angiographic restenosis occurring in regions treated with a PES but also developing in gaps segments between PES and in BMS that were placed in as bailout to PES. These findings underscore the need for meticulous technique for the placement of DES for in-stent restenosis with coverage of all regions of balloon injury with PES.

TAXUS-IV

The TAXUS-IV trial randomly assigned 1314 patients with complex, native coronary stenoses to treatment with BMS or SR PES [44]. Similar to the SIRIUS trial, patients enrolled in the TAXUS-IV study had complex lesions that were between 10 and 28 mm in length and located in vessels with a diameter between 2.5 and 3.75 mm. The frequency of diabetes mellitus (24.2%), reference vessel diameter (2.75 mm) mean lesion length (13.4 mm), and stent length (21.8 mm) were similar in the two treatment groups, and comparable to the lesion characteristics in patients enrolled in the SIRIUS trial. The primary study endpoint, 9-month target vessel revascularization (TVR), was reduced from 12.0% in patients assigned to BMS to 4.7% in patients assigned to PES ($P < .001$). TLR occurred in 11.3% of patients in the BMS group and in 3.0% of patients in the PES group ($P < .001$). The 9-month composite rates of death from cardiac causes or MI (4.7% and 4.3%, respectively) and stent thrombosis (0.6% and 0.8%, respectively) were similar in the group that received a paclitaxel-eluting stent and the group that received a bare metal stent. The reductions in TLR and MACE were sustained 1 year after the procedure [50].

Nine-month angiographic follow-up was performed in 732 patients and demonstrated a reduction from 0.92 ± 0.58 mm in patients treated with BMS to 0.39 ± 0.50 in patients treated with a TAXUS stent ($P < .001$). Binary angiographic restenosis, defined as a greater than 50% diameter follow-up stenosis, occurred in 26.6% of patients with BMS and 7.9% of patients with PES ($P < .001$). An IVUS substudy analysis in 170 patients found a uniform suppression of intimal hyperplasia along the length of the stent, with reduction in neointimal volume in patients treated with the TAXUS stent (18 ± 18 mm^3) compared with patient treated with a BMS (41 ± 23 mm^3, $P < .001$) [51]. Incomplete stent apposition at 9 months was similar in patients treated with the TAXUS stent (3.0%) and those treated with BMS (4.0%, $P = .12$).

TAXUS-V

The TAXUS-V trial was designed to evaluate the angiographic and clinical outcomes of 1156 patients with very complex lesions who were treated with SR PES or BMS [52]. Patients in this study were required to have native coronary stenoses in vessel diameters between 2.25 and 4.0 mm and lesion lengths between 10 and 46 mm and multiple stents. The vessel diameter (2.69 ± 0.57 mm), lesion lengths (17.2 ± 9.2 mm), and stent lengths per lesion (1.38 ± 0.58 mm) indicated a more complex subset of patients. The primary endpoint, 9-month TVR, was reduced from 17.3% in patients assigned to BMS to 12.1% in those assigned to PES ($P < .001$). The rates of death and MI were similar in both groups. Angiographic restenosis was reduced from 33.9% in those treated with BMS to 18.9% in patients assigned to

treatment with PES ($P < .001$). Patients treated with 2.25 mm stents had a lower rate of angiographic restenosis with PES (31.2%) than those treated with BMS (49.4%, $P = .01$). Although this study demonstrated a reduction in events associated with the use of PES over BMS, the overall higher event rate in these patients suggested that further improvements in clinical outcomes could be obtained.

TAXUS-VI

The TAXUS-VI trial was designed to evaluate clinical and angiographic outcomes in 448 patients with complex, long stenoses who were assigned randomly to treatment with one or more MR PES or BMS [53]. The primary endpoint of the study, 9-month TVR, was reduced by 53% from 19.4% in patients assigned to BMS to 9.1% of patients assigned PES ($P = .0027$). In-stent angiographic restenosis also was reduced from 32.9% in the patients assigned to treatment with BMS to 9.1% in the patients assigned to treatment with PES ($P < .0001$). TLR was reduced from 18.9% in patients assigned to treatment with BMS to 6.8% in patients assigned to treatment with PES ($P = .0001$).

TAXUS registries and subset analyses

The TAXUS stent is also effective in reducing the angiographic and clinical recurrence in diabetic patients. Medically treated diabetes was present in 318 (24%) of the 1314 patients enrolled in the TAXUS-IV trial; of these, 105 patients required insulin therapy [54]. Diabetic patients treated with the PES stent had an 81% lower rate of 9-month binary angiographic restenosis (6.4%) than patients treated with BMS (34.5%, $P < .0001$). Diabetic patients also had a 65% lower rate of 12-month TLR (7.4%) than patients treated with a bare metal stent (20.9%, $P = .0008$). Insulin-requiring diabetic patients assigned to treatment with PES had an 82% lower angiographic restenosis rate (7.7%) than patients assigned to treatment with BMS (42.9%, $P = .0065$). Similarly, 1-year TLR rates were lowered by 68% in insulin-requiring patients assigned to treatment with a TAXUS stent (6.2% versus 19.4% in BMS-assigned patients, $P = .07$). There were no differences in the occurrence of death or MI in the two groups.

The TAXUS trials have demonstrated specific benefits in women [55] and in patients who have acute coronary syndromes [56], including ST segment elevation MI [57,58], saphenous vein graft disease [59], left anterior descending artery stenoses [60], bifurcation lesions [61], chronic total occlusion [62], and in those undergoing direct stenting [63].

Randomized comparisons of sirolimus-eluting stents and paclitaxel-eluting stent

A series of randomized studies has provided head-to-head comparisons of the SES and PES in various complex lesions subsets. Although patients in these trials were assigned randomly to treatment with PES or SES, they have varied with the frequency of angiographic follow-up, angiographic methodology used for the analysis, and the methods used for adjudication of clinical events. Given the impact of the oculostenotic reflex on the occurrence of late revascularizations, studies that have had rigorous event adjudication with sufficient sample sizes to justify the conclusions take precedent over smaller ones with less rigorously defined endpoints.

REALITY

The REALITY trial was a prospective, randomized clinical trial performed at 90 hospitals in Europe, Latin America, and Asia that included 1386 patients with one or two de novo lesions in small (2.25 to 3.00 mm) caliper vessels who were randomized to treatment with a SES or PES [64]. Diabetes mellitus was present in 28.0% of patients, The primary endpoint, 8-month in-lesion binary restenosis, occurred in 9.6% of patients assigned to treatment with SES and 11.1% of patients assigned to treatment with PES (RR 0.84, $P = .31$), despite a lower in-stent late loss in patients assigned to treatment with SES (0.09 mm) than in those assigned to treatment with PES (0.31 mm, $P < .001$). Patients treated with SES and PES had similar 1-year frequencies of MACE (10.7% in SES patients and 11.4% in PES patients, $P = .73$) and TLR (6.0% in SES and 6.1% in PES, $P > .99$). The results of this study suggested that the beneficial effects on intimal hyperplasia observed with SES did not translate into beneficial effects on clinical outcomes. The frequency of binary (and clinical restenosis) appears related to the standard deviation of the late lumen loss measurement and the rightward skewedness of the distribution histogram rather than to the absolute value of late lumen loss alone [65].

SIRTAX

The SIRTAX trial, a trial of 1012 patients who were assigned randomly to treatment with SES or PES evaluated all comers to the catheterization laboratory [66]. The primary study endpoint, a composite of 9-month MACE, occurred in 6.2% of patients in the SES group and 10.8% of patients in the PES group (hazard ratio [HR] 0.56, $P = .009$), primarily because of reductions in TLR in patients assigned to treatment with SES (4.8% versus 8.3% in patients in the PES group, $P = .03$). There were no differences in death, MI, or subacute stent thrombosis in the two groups. The binary angiographic restenosis rate in the 53.4% of patients with angiographic follow-up was 6.6% in patients treated with SES and 11.7% in patients treated with PES ($P = .02$).

ISAR-Diabetes

In the ISAR-Diabetes trial, 250 diabetic patients were assigned randomly to treatment with PES or SES. The primary study endpoint, in-segment late luminal loss, was segment restenosis (at least 50% diameter stenosis) occurred in 16.5% of the PES patients and in 6.9% of the SES patients ($P = .03$). TLR was required in 12.0% of the PES patients and in 6.4% of the SES patients ($P = .13$).

TAXI trial

In a smaller series, 202 patients were assigned randomly to treatment with a PES or SES [67]. The incidence of late (mean 7 month) MACE was 4% with the PES and 6% with the SES ($P = .8$). Similarly, the need for target lesion revascularization was very low in both groups (1% with PES and 3% with SES).

ISAR-DESIRE

The ISAR-DESIRE study was a study of the effect of balloon angioplasty, SES, or PES in 300 patients with angiographically significant in-stent restenosis [68]. The primary endpoint, 6-month in-segment angiographic restenosis, was 44.6% in the balloon angioplasty group, 14.3% in the SES group ($P < .001$ versus balloon angioplasty), and 21.7% in the PES group ($P = .001$ versus balloon angioplasty) [68]. The incidence of target vessel revascularization was 33.0% in the balloon angioplasty group, 8.0% in the SES group ($P < .001$ versus balloon angioplasty), and 19.0% in the PES group ($P = .02$ versus balloon angioplasty)

[68]. There was a trend for better outcomes in patients treated with SES compared with PES.

Meta-analyses of comparative trials

In aggregate, many of the comparative studies were too small to make definitive conclusions about the comparative benefit of SES or PES stents. A subsequent meta-analysis compared the clinical and angiographic outcomes of SES and PES in six randomized head-to-head clinical trials that included 3669 patients [69]. TLR occurred less often in patients treated with SES (5.1%) compared with PES (7.8%) ($P = .001$). Angiographic restenosis occurred less often in patients assigned to SES (9.3%) compared with PES (13.1%) ($P = .001$). Event rates were similar with SES and PES for stent thrombosis (SES 0.9%, PES 1.1%, $P = .62$), death (1.4% and 1.6%, respectively; $P = .56$), and the composite of death and MI (4.9% and 5.8%, respectively; $P = .23$). Although this meta-analysis suggests restenosis superiority of SES over PES, it needs to be viewed in the context of the variable endpoints, sample size, and adjudication processes that were used to formulate the analysis. Larger randomized clinical trials will be useful in providing additional analyses for the comparative studies.

Other ongoing drug-eluting stents programs

Endeavor

The Endeavor stent (Medtronic, Minneapolis, Minnesota) uses a cobalt chromium stent platform, a durable, antithrombotic, phoshorylcholine (PC)-encapsulated coating, and another G1 cell cycle inhibitor, zotarolimus, which elutes from the PC coating over several days [70]. Cobalt chromium alloys provide the potential for being stronger than stainless steel with a higher density that allows for similar radiopacity with thinner (0.0036") stent filaments. The potential advantage of phosphorylcholine is that it lessens platelet adhesion to the metal surface, and is noninflammatory on long-term vascular compatibility studies. Zotarolimus delivered in this manner reduced intimal hyperplasia by up to 40% in a porcine model of stent injury [71].

The Endeavor I study was the first clinical study to evaluate the safety and feasibility of the Endeavor stent system for treating symptomatic coronary artery disease. It enrolled 100 patients at eight centers in Australia and New Zealand [70].

The procedure and device deployment success rates were 100%. At 12 months, in-stent late lumen loss was 0.61 ± 0.44 mm; in-segment late lumen loss was 0.43 ± 0.44 mm, and neointimal hyperplasia volume was 14.2 ± 11.8 mm^3 (corresponding to a percent volume obstruction of $9.7\% \pm 8.5\%$). The binary angiographic restenosis rates at 4 and 12 months were 2.1% and 5.4%, respectively, and the pattern of neointimal hyperplasia was greatest within the stent and not at the stent edges. The cumulative incidence of MACE was 1% at 30 days and 2% at 4 and 12 months.

The Endeavor-II trial enrolled 1197 patients who had a single coronary stenosis in a vessel diameter between 2.25 and 3.50 mm and a lesion length between 14 and 27 mm. Patients were assigned randomly to receive an Endeavor stent or BMS [72]. Patients were included with complex coronary disease similar to the SIRIUS and TAXUS-IV studies, including the presence of diabetes (20.1%), smaller vessel diameters (2.75 mm), and longer lesions (lesion length, 14.2 mm). The primary endpoint of 9-month target vessel failure was reduced from 15.1% with BMS to 8.00% with the Endeavor stent ($P < .0005$). The rate of MACE was reduced from 14.4% with BMS to 7.3% with the Endeavor stent ($P < .0005$). TLR was 4.6% with Endeavor stent compared with 11.8% with BMS ($P < .005$). The rate of stent thrombosis was 0.5% with the Endeavor ABT drug-eluting stent, not different from 1.2% with bare metal stent. In-stent late loss was reduced from 1.03 ± 0.59 to 0.62 ± 0.47 ($P < .0001$), and in-segment late loss was reduced from 0.71 ± 0.61 to 0.36 ± 0.47 ($P < .0001$), with the Endeavor ABT drug-eluting stent. The rate of in-segment angiographic binary restenosis was reduced from 35.0% to 13.7% with the Endeavor stent ($P < .0001$). There was no evidence for edge stenosis, coronary aneurysm formation, or late acquired malposition by intravascular ultrasound imaging. The Endeavor III trial compared patients treated with SES and an Endeavor stent, and the Endeavor IV trial will compare patients treated with PES and an Endeavor stent.

The PISCES program

The Conor stent (Conor Medsystems, Menlo Park, California) is comprised of intrastrut wells with an erodable polymer that is designed specifically for drug delivery with programmable pharmacokinetics [73]. The PISCES-I study included 244 patients who were treated with a bare metal Conor stent or one of six different release formulations that varied in dose (10 or 30 µg) and elution release kinetics, direction, and duration (5, 10, and 30 days) [73]. The lowest in-stent late loss (0.38 mm, $P < .01$; and 0.30 mm, $P < .01$) and volume obstruction (8%, $P < .01$; and 5%, $P < 0.01$) were observed with the 10 and 30 µg doses in the 30-day release groups respectively, whereas the highest in-stent late loss (0.88 mm), volume obstruction (26%), and restenosis rate (11.6%) were observed in the BMS group [73]. This stent is being evaluated in a randomized study compared with the TAXUS stent.

Everolimus-eluting durable polymer stent

The Xience stent (Guidant Corporation, Santa Clara, California) is comprised of the Vision cobalt chromium stent (Guidant Corp., Japan), a durable polymer coating, and everolimus, a sirolimus analog that has immunosuppressive and antiproliferative effects. This SPIRIT-First was a first-in-man single blind randomized trial that compared the safety and efficacy of the Xience stent with BMS in 56 patients who had de novo coronary lesions [74]. The in-stent late loss and percentage diameter stenosis at 1 year were 0.24 mm and 18%, respectively, in the Xience group and 0.84 mm and 37% in the BMS group ($P < .001$). Significantly less neointimal hyperplasia was observed in patients treated with the Xience stent (neointimal volume obstruction, 10% $\pm$ 7% versus 28% $\pm$ 12% in patients treated with BMS, $P < .001$). The overall MACE rate was 15.4% in the everolimus arm and 21.4% in the bare stent arm.

SPIRIT II is a 300-patient prospective, single blind, European, randomized noninferiority trial comparing the Xience stent with the TAXUS paclitaxel-eluting stent in patients who have native coronary artery disease. SPIRIT III is a 1380-patient global clinical trial evaluating the Xience Stent. It will include randomization in 1002 patients who will receive either the Xience stent or PES. Recruitment for this trial has been completed.

Biolimus A-9-eluting stent

The Stealth drug eluting stent program (Biosensors, Singapore) includes the balloon-expandable S stent, a bioresorbable polymer coating, and Biolimus A-9, a sirolimus analog with potent inhibition of intimal hyperplasia. A randomized pilot study in 42 patients using everolimus rather than Biolimus A-9 compared with a BMS found a low in-stent late lumen loss (0.10 $\pm$ 0.22 mm compared with 0.85 $\pm$ 0.32 mm in patients treated with a BMS, $P < .0001$) [75]. There was no in-stent restenoses in patients treated with an everolimus-eluting stent. A larger multi-center trial with the Stealth stent is planned in the United States.

Failed or minimally effective drug-eluting stent programs

Actinomycin-D-eluting stent

The ACTinomycin-eluting stent Improves Outcomes by reducing Neointimal hyperplasia (ACTION) trial randomly assigned 360 patients to receive an actinomycin-eluting stent (AES) stent that eluted 2.5 or 10 µg/cm^2 of actinomycin D or BMS [76]. The in-stent late lumen loss and the proximal and distal edges were higher in both AES groups than in the BMS group and resulted in higher 6-month and 1-year MACE (34.8% and 43.1% in the 2.5 and 10 µg/cm^2 group versus 13.5% in the BMS group), driven exclusively by TLR without excess death or myocardial infarction.

Paclitaxel spray stents

Three trials have evaluated the benefit of the delivery of a spray coating of paclitaxel that elutes from the stent over 24 to 48 hours. The ASPECT trial randomly assigned 177 patients to treatment with low-dose paclitaxel (3.1 µ/mm^2), high-dose paclitaxel (3.1 µ/mm^2), or BMS [77,78]. Patients treated with high-dose paclitaxel had a significantly lower binary restenosis rate than control-treated patients (4% versus 27%, $P < .001$) [77]. There was a stepwise reduction in intimal hyperplasia within the stented segment in patients who were treated with high-dose paclitaxel [77].

In the European evaLUation of the pacliTaxel Eluting Stent (ELUTES) pilot clinical trial, the safety and efficacy of the V-Flex Plus (Cook Group Inc., Bloomington, Indiana) coronary stents that were spray coated on the abluminal surface with escalating doses of paclitaxel were evaluated [79]. Binary angiographic restenosis decreased from 20.6% in the lowest dose paclitaxel group to 3.2% in the highest paclitaxel dose group ($P = .056$).

The DELIVER trial was a larger randomized, multi-center clinical evaluation that evaluated the nonpolymer-based paclitaxel-coated stent compared with BMS in 1043 patients who had focal de novo coronary lesions [80]. Although in-stent late lumen loss was lower with the DELIVER stent (0.81 mm versus 0.98 mm for BMS, $P = .003$), there we no significant differences in the primary study endpoint in patients treated with DELIVER (11.9%) and BMS (14.5%; $P = .12$). These findings suggest that the release kinetics may be an important determinant in the delivery of paclitaxel.

Paclitaxel derivative-eluting polymeric sleeve

A multi-sleeve drug delivery coronary stent (QuaDS-QP-2, Boston Scientific) contained up to 4000 μg of a taxol-derived lipophilic microtubule inhibitor (QP2) designed to delivery high quantities of drug to the vessel wall. Following a pilot study in 32 patients showing a low degree of intimal hyperplasia [81], the Study to COmpare REstenosis rate between QueST and QuaDS-QP2 (SCORE) trial was performed to compare the 7-hexanoyltaxol (QP2)-eluting stents (qDES) with BMS in 266 patients [82]. The qDES showed a 68% reduction in neointimal growth within the stent ($P < .0001$) and a significantly lower angiographic restenosis rate with the qDES (6.4% versus 36.9% in BMS patients, $P < .001$). The program was terminated, however, because of an unacceptable 10.2% subacute stent thrombosis rate [82] and delayed restenosis 12 months after the procedure [83], potentially because of the non-reabsorbable polymer alone, which may have induced chronic inflammation [84].

Outstanding issues

The use of DES has reduced the occurrence of restenosis after stent placement dramatically, but numerous potential issues have been addressed incompletely from current clinical data, primarily related to the lingering issue of stent thrombosis, the infrequent occurrence of stent restenosis, and the cost-effectiveness of the DES.

Early stent thrombosis

There does not appear to be an increased propensity for early (30 days to 12 months) stent thrombosis when patients are treated with extended dual antiplatelet therapy with SES (2 to 3 months of antiplatelet therapy) or PES (6 months of antiplatelet therapy) compared with BMS [85].

In an analysis of 2512 patients treated with BMS, SES, or PES, there were no differences in stent thrombosis among the three stents [86]. Bifurcation stenting in the setting of acute MI was an independent risk factor for angiographic ST in the entire population ($P < .001$). Stent thrombosis was associated with a 30-day mortality of 15% and a nonfatal MI rate of 60% [86].

Two meta-analyses confirmed the absence of early incremental risk for stent thrombosis associated with the use of DES over BMS. A meta-analysis of 3817 patients that reviewed eight randomized trials compared the stent thrombosis rate in patients treated with BMS and PES and found no incremental risk with PES within 12 months after stent placement [85]. Another meta-analysis of 10 randomized trials that included 5066 patients followed for 6 to 12 months after the procedure found no major differences in the stent thrombosis rate between SES and BMS [87].

In contrast to patients taking the prescribed duration of dual antiplatelet therapy, premature discontinuation of dual antiplatelet therapy is associated with a higher rate of stent thrombosis [88–90]. In a prospective observational cohort study of 2229 consecutive patients who underwent successful implantation of SES or PES, aspirin was continued indefinitely and clopidogrel or ticlopidine for at least 3 months after sirolimus-eluting and for at least 6 months after paclitaxel-eluting stent implantation [90]. Stent thrombosis occurred in 1.3% of patients by 9-month follow-up, resulting in a high (45%) mortality rate. Predictors of stent thrombosis included premature discontinuation of antiplatelet therapy (HR, 89.8, $P < .001$), renal failure (HR, 6.49, $P < .001$), bifurcation lesions (HR, 6.42, $P < .001$), diabetes (HR, 3.71, $P = .001$), and a lower ejection fraction (HR, 1.09, $P < .001$ for each 10% decrease). These findings have important implications for patients undergoing noncardiac surgery within the first 3 to 6 months after DES placement.

Late stent thrombosis

With the accumulation of longer-term follow-up with patients undergoing treatment with DES, there has been the identification of a small number of patients who develop stent thrombosis late (greater than 30 to 180 days) following DES placement, most commonly following the discontinuation aspirin or clopidogrel. These events have occurred with both SES and PER [91–93]. In a registry of 2006 patients treated with either

PES or SES, late angiographic stent thrombosis, defined as angiographically proven stent thrombosis associated with acute symptoms more than 30 days (average duration of follow-up, 1.5 years), there were eight angiographically confirmed stent thromboses in eight patients [91], including three patients treated with SES (at 2, 25, and 26 months) and five patients treated with PES (at 6, 7, 8, 11, and 14.5 months) [91]. The development of stent thromboses appeared to be related to discontinuation of dual antiplatelet therapy after DES placement. The potential for developing late stent thrombosis appears related to delayed endothelialization of the stent [94] or an inflammatory reaction to the durable polymer coating [84,95,96] and delayed healing [97].

The effect of late-acquired incomplete stent apposition on stent thrombosis has not been demonstrated in late outcome studies. Repeat coronary arteriography and IVUS performed on 13 patients who received SES and showed incomplete stent apposition at 6 months found no further vascular remodeling was observed in the vessel segment with incomplete stent apposition [10]. In the TAXUS-II trial, predictive factors of late-acquired incomplete stent apposition (ISA) were lesion length, unstable angina, and absence of diabetes. No stent thrombosis occurred in the patients diagnosed with ISA over a period of 12 months [98].

Predictors of restenosis after drug-eluting stents

Although clinical restenosis is an uncommon finding after DES placement, numerous factors contribute to its occurrence, including lesion length, stent length, vessel diameter, the presence of diabetes, and underexpansion of the DES [99–101]. In an angiographic substudy of SIRIUS, a multiple regression model predicting late angiographic outcome found that the stented lesion length and excess stent length were associated with absolute increases in late lumen renarrowing [100]. Delayed healing within the vessel wall with DES may predispose to late aneurysm formation, and isolated aneurysms have been reported with SES [102,103] and PES [104].

Cost-effectiveness of drug-eluting stents

With the initial introduction of DES, there was concern that the increase in price and quantity of stents used during PCI would have a detrimental impact on hospital budgets and overall resource allocation [105]. It was appreciated that DES reduced the morbidity associated with restenosis, but had little effect on the overall mortality of patients undergoing revascularization. As a result, cost-effectiveness studies were needed to appropriately weigh the expenditures associated with the use of DES with other potentially more effective morbidity and mortality reducing therapies. In the RAVEL trial, medical costs were tracked in 238 patients for 1 year after the procedure using resource allocation and Dutch unit cost methods [106]. The higher initial procedural costs associated with the use of SES were nearly offset by cost savings that occurred after the procedure because of reductions in the need for repeat revascularizations in those assigned to SES. A similar cost and resource allocation analysis was performed in patients enrolled in the SIRIUS trial that included 1058 patients with complex coronary stenoses assigned to PCI with SES or BMS [107]. Although the initial hospital costs increased by $2881 per patient in those assigned to SES, the follow-up costs were reduced by $2571 dollars per patient in those assigned to SES, mostly because of reduction in the need for TLR. Accordingly, the incremental cost-effectiveness ratio for SES was $1650 dollars per repeat revascularization event avoided or $27,540 per quality adjusted year of life gained. These savings become even more profound as the prices of DES fall with increased availability and competition. Ongoing studies will evaluate the cost benefit of DES or CABG in patients with multi-vessel disease.

Drug-eluting stents have become an integral component of PCI in patients with single and multi-vessel coronary artery disease. The dramatic reductions in 1-year clinical events associated with the use of DES have been sustained with late follow-up studies, albeit at the expense of a small (0.4%) incidence of late stent thrombosis that occurs up to 3 years after the procedure. Future generations of DES will include the development of more deliverable stents using unique metallic alloys, likely elimination of the durable polymer coating in favor of bioresorbable ones, and the development of antithrombotic agents that will reduce the risk of late thrombosis. Ongoing studies will evaluate the benefit of DES over coronary bypass surgery in patients who have multi-vessel disease, including those who have diabetes mellitus.

References

[1] Altmann DB, Racz M, Battleman DS, et al. Reduction in angioplasty complications after the

introduction of coronary stents: results from a consecutive series of 2242 patients. Am Heart J 1996; 132(3):503–7.

[2] Serruys PW, de Jaegere P, Kiemeneij F, et al. A comparison of balloon-expandable stent implantation with balloon angioplasty in patients with coronary artery disease. Benestent Study Group. N Engl J Med 1994;331(8):489–95.

[3] Fischman DL, Leon MB, Baim DS, et al. A randomized comparison of coronary stent placement and balloon angioplasty in the treatment of coronary artery disease. Stent Restenosis Study Investigators. N Engl J Med 1994;331(8):496–501.

[4] Baim D, Cutlip D, Midei M, et al. Final results of a randomized trial comparing the MULTI-LINK stent with the Palmaz-Schatz stent for narrowings in native coronary arteries. Am J Cardiol 2001; 87(2):157–62.

[5] Heuser R, Lopez A, Kuntz R, et al. SMART: The microstent's ability to limit restenosis trial. Catheter Cardiovasc Interv 2001;52(3):269–77 [discussion 278].

[6] Baim D, Cutlip D, O'Shaughnessy C, et al. Final results of a randomized trial comparing the NIR stent to the Palmaz-Schatz stent for narrowings in native coronary arteries. Am J Cardiol 2001;87(2):152–6.

[7] Cutlip D, Chauhan M, Baim D, et al. Clinical restenosis after coronary stenting: perspectives from multicenter clinical trials. J Am Coll Cardiol 2002;40(12):2082–9.

[8] Moses J, Leon M, Popma J, et al. Sirolimus-eluting stents versus standard stents in patients with stenosis in a native coronary artery. N Engl J Med 2003; 349(14):1315–23.

[9] Sousa J, Costa M, Abizaid A, et al. Sustained suppression of neointimal proliferation by sirolimus-eluting stents: one-year angiographic and intravascular ultrasound follow-up. Circulation 2001;104(17):2007–11.

[10] Degertekin M, Serruys P, Tanabe K, et al. Long-term follow-up of incomplete stent apposition in patients who received sirolimus-eluting stent for de novo coronary lesions: an intravascular ultrasound analysis. Circulation 2003;108(22): 2747–50.

[11] Sousa J, Costa M, Abizaid A, et al. Four-year angiographic and intravascular ultrasound follow-up of patients treated with sirolimus-eluting stents. Circulation 2005;111(18):2326–9.

[12] Sousa JE, Costa MA, Abizaid A, et al. Lack of neointimal proliferation after implantation of sirolimus-coated stents in human coronary arteries: a quantitative coronary angiography and three-dimensional intravascular ultrasound study. Circulation 2001; 103(2):192–5.

[13] Sousa J, Costa M, Sousa A, et al. Two-year angiographic and intravascular ultrasound follow-up after implantation of sirolimus-eluting stents in human coronary arteries. Circulation 2003;107(3):381–3.

[14] Morice M, Serruys P, Sousa J, et al. A randomized comparison of a sirolimus-eluting stent with a standard stent for coronary revascularization. N Engl J Med 2002;346(23):1773–80.

[15] Regar E, Serruys P, Bode C, et al. Angiographic findings of the multi-center Randomized Study With the Sirolimus-Eluting Bx Velocity Balloon-Expandable Stent (RAVEL): sirolimus-eluting stents inhibit restenosis irrespective of the vessel size. Circulation 2002;106(15):1949–56.

[16] Tanabe K, Serruys P, Degertekin M, et al. Fate of side branches after coronary arterial sirolimus-eluting stent implantation. Am J Cardiol 2002;90(9):937–41.

[17] Serruys P, Degertekin M, Tanabe K, et al. Intravascular ultrasound findings in the multi-center, randomized, double-blind RAVEL (RAndomized study with the sirolimus-eluting VElocity balloon-expandable stent in the treatment of patients with de novo native coronary artery Lesions) trial. Circulation 2002;106(7):798–803.

[18] Fajadet J, Morice M, Bode C, et al. Maintenance of long-term clinical benefit with sirolimus-eluting coronary stents: three-year results of the RAVEL trial. Circulation 2005;111(8):1040–4.

[19] Holmes D, Leon M, Moses J, et al. Analysis of 1-year clinical outcomes in the SIRIUS trial: a randomized trial of a sirolimus-eluting stent versus a standard stent in patients at high risk for coronary restenosis. Circulation 2004;109(5):634–40.

[20] Popma J, Leon M, Moses J, et al. Quantitative assessment of angiographic restenosis after sirolimus-eluting stent implantation in native coronary arteries. Circulation 2004;110(25):3773–80.

[21] Schofer J, Schluter M, Gershlick A, et al. Sirolimus-eluting stents for treatment of patients with long atherosclerotic lesions in small coronary arteries: double-blind, randomised controlled trial (E-SIRIUS). Lancet 2003;362(9390):1093–9.

[22] Schampaert E, Cohen E, Schluter M, et al. The Canadian study of the sirolimus-eluting stent in the treatment of patients with long de novo lesions in small native coronary arteries (C-SIRIUS). J Am Coll Cardiol 2004;43(6):1110–5.

[23] Sousa J, Costa M, Abizaid A, et al. Sirolimus-eluting stent for the treatment of in-stent restenosis: a quantitative coronary angiography and three-dimensional intravascular ultrasound study. Circulation 2003;107(1):24–7.

[24] Airoldi F, Rogacka R, Briguori C, et al. Comparison of clinical and angiographic outcome of sirolimus-eluting stent implantation versus cutting balloon angioplasty for coronary in-stent restenosis. Am J Cardiol 2004;94(10):1297–300.

[25] Saia F, Lemos P, Hoye A, et al. Clinical outcomes for sirolimus-eluting stent implantation and vascular brachytherapy for the treatment of in-stent restenosis. Catheter Cardiovasc Interv 2004;62(3):283–8.

[26] Degertekin M, Regar E, Tanabe K, et al. Sirolimus-eluting stent for treatment of complex in-stent

restenosis. The first clinical experience. J Am Coll Cardiol 2003;41(2):184–9.

[27] Holmes D, Popma J, Kuntz R, et al. A multi-center, randomized study of the sirolimus-eluting Bx velocity stent versus intravascular brachytherapy in the treatment of patients with in-stent restenosis in native coronary arteries. Late-breaking clinical trials. Dallas (TX): American Heart Association; 2005.

[28] Lemos P, Lee C, Degertekin M, et al. Early outcome after sirolimus-eluting stent implantation in patients with acute coronary syndromes: insights from the Rapamycin-Eluting Stent Evaluated At Rotterdam Cardiology Hospital (RESEARCH) registry. J Am Coll Cardiol 2003;41(11):2093–9.

[29] Lemos P, Saia F, Hofma S, et al. Short- and long-term clinical benefit of sirolimus-eluting stents compared to conventional bare stents for patients with acute myocardial infarction. J Am Coll Cardiol 2004;43(4):704–8.

[30] Moussa I, Leon M, Baim D, et al. Impact of sirolimus-eluting stents on outcome in diabetic patients: a SIRIUS (SIRolImUS-coated Bx Velocity balloon-expandable stent in the treatment of patients with de novo coronary artery lesions) substudy. Circulation 2004;109(19):2273–8.

[31] Ardissino D, Cavallini C, Bramucci E, et al. Sirolimus-eluting vs uncoated stents for prevention of restenosis in small coronary arteries: a randomized trial. JAMA 2004;292(22):2727–34.

[32] Hoye A, Tanabe K, Lemos P, et al. Significant reduction in restenosis after the use of sirolimus-eluting stents in the treatment of chronic total occlusions. J Am Coll Cardiol 2004;43(11):1954–8.

[33] Hoye A, Lemos P, Arampatzis C, et al. Effectiveness of the sirolimus-eluting stent in the treatment of patients with a prior history of coronary artery bypass graft surgery. Coron Artery Dis 2004;15(3):171–5.

[34] Price M, Sawhney N, Kao J, et al. Clinical outcomes after sirolimus-eluting stent implantation for de novo saphenous vein graft lesions. Catheter Cardiovasc Interv 2005;65(2):208–11.

[35] Valgimigli M, van MC, Ong A, et al. Short- and long-term clinical outcome after drug-eluting stent implantation for the percutaneous treatment of left main coronary artery disease: insights from the Rapamycin-Eluting and Taxus Stent Evaluated At Rotterdam Cardiology Hospital registries (RESEARCH and T-SEARCH). Circulation 2005; 111(11):1383–9.

[36] Park S, Kim Y, Lee B, et al. Sirolimus-eluting stent implantation for unprotected left main coronary artery stenosis: comparison with bare metal stent implantation. J Am Coll Cardiol 2005;45(3):351–6.

[37] Aoki J, Hoye A, Staferov A, et al. Sirolimus-eluting stent implantation for chronic total occlusion of the left main coronary artery. J Interv Cardiol 2005; 18(1):65–9.

[38] Arampatzis C, Lemos P, Tanabe K, et al. Effectiveness of sirolimus-eluting stent for treatment of left main coronary artery disease. Am J Cardiol 2003; 92(3):327–9.

[39] Daemen J, Lemos P, Serruys P. Multi-lesion culotte and crush bifurcation stenting with sirolimus-eluting stents: long-term angiographic outcome. J Invasive Cardiol 2003;15(11):653–6.

[40] Colombo A, Moses J, Morice M, et al. Randomized study to evaluate sirolimus-eluting stents implanted at coronary bifurcation lesions. Circulation 2004;109(10):1244–9.

[41] Rizik D, Dowler D, Villegas B. Balloon alignment T-stenting for bifurcation coronary artery disease using the sirolimus-eluting stent. J Invasive Cardiol 2005;17(8):437–9.

[42] Iakovou I, Sangiorgi G, Stankovic G, et al. Results and follow-up after implantation of four or more sirolimus-eluting stents in the same patient. Catheter Cardiovasc Interv 2005;64(4):436–9 [discussion 440–1].

[43] Schluter M, Schofer J, Gershlick A, et al. Direct stenting of native de novo coronary artery lesions with the sirolimus-eluting stent: a post hoc subanalysis of the pooled E- and C-SIRIUS trials. J Am Coll Cardiol 2005;45(1):10–3.

[44] Stone G, Ellis S, Cox D, et al. A polymer-based, paclitaxel-eluting stent in patients with coronary artery disease. N Engl J Med 2004;350(3):221–31.

[45] Grube E, Silber S, Hauptmann K, et al. TAXUS I: six- and twelve-month results from a randomized, double-blind trial on a slow-release paclitaxel-eluting stent for de novo coronary lesions. Circulation 2003;107(1):38–42.

[46] Grube E, Silber S, Hauptmann K, et al. Two-year-plus follow-up of a paclitaxel-eluting stent in de novo coronary narrowings (TAXUS I). Am J Cardiol 2005;96(1):79–82.

[47] Colombo A, Drzewiecki J, Banning A, et al. Randomized study to assess the effectiveness of slow- and moderate-release polymer-based Paclitaxel-eluting stents for coronary artery lesions. Circulation 2003;108(7):788–94.

[48] Serruys P, Degertekin M, Tanabe K, et al. Vascular responses at proximal and distal edges of paclitaxel-eluting stents: serial intravascular ultrasound analysis from the TAXUS II trial. Circulation 2004;109(5):627–33.

[49] Tanabe K, Serruys P, Grube E, et al. TAXUS III trial: in-stent restenosis treated with stent-based delivery of paclitaxel incorporated in a slow-release polymer formulation. Circulation 2003;107(4): 559–64.

[50] Stone G, Ellis S, Cox D, et al. One-year clinical results with the slow-release, polymer-based, paclitaxel-eluting TAXUS stent: the TAXUS-IV trial. Circulation 2004;109(16):1942–7.

[51] Cheneau E, Pichard A, Satler L, et al. Intravascular ultrasound stent area of sirolimus-eluting stents and its impact on late outcome. Am J Cardiol 2005;95(10):1240–2.

[52] Stone G, Ellis S, Cannon L, et al. Comparison of a polymer-based paclitaxel-eluting stent with a bare metal stent in patients with complex coronary artery disease: a randomized controlled trial. JAMA 2005;294(10):1215–23.

[53] Dawkins K, Grube E, Guagliumi G, et al. Clinical efficacy of polymer-based paclitaxel-eluting stents in the treatment of complex, long coronary artery lesions from a multi-center, randomized trial: support for the use of drug-eluting stents in contemporary clinical practice. Circulation 2005;112(21):3306–13.

[54] Hermiller J, Raizner A, Cannon L, et al. Outcomes with the polymer-based paclitaxel-eluting TAXUS stent in patients with diabetes mellitus: the TAXUS-IV trial. J Am Coll Cardiol 2005;45(8):1172–9.

[55] Lansky A, Costa R, Mooney M, et al. Gender-based outcomes after paclitaxel-eluting stent implantation in patients with coronary artery disease. J Am Coll Cardiol 2005;45(8):1180–5.

[56] Moses J, Mehran R, Nikolsky E, et al. Outcomes with the paclitaxel-eluting stent in patients with acute coronary syndromes: analysis from the TAXUS-IV trial. J Am Coll Cardiol 2005;45(8): 1165–71.

[57] Valgimigli M, Percoco G, Cicchitelli G, et al. High-dose bolus tirofiban and sirolimus eluting stent versus abiciximab and bare metal stent in acute myocardial infarction (STRATEGY) study–protocol design and demography of the first 100 patients. Cardiovasc Drugs Ther 2004;18(3):225–30.

[58] Valgimigli M, Percoco G, Malagutti P, et al. Tirofiban and sirolimus-eluting stent vs abciximab and bare-metal stent for acute myocardial infarction: a randomized trial. JAMA 2005;293(17): 2109–17.

[59] Tsuchida K, Ong A, Aoki J, et al. Immediate and one-year outcome of percutaneous intervention of saphenous vein graft disease with paclitaxel-eluting stents. Am J Cardiol 2005;96(3):395–8.

[60] Dangas G, Ellis S, Shlofmitz R, et al. Outcomes of paclitaxel-eluting stent implantation in patients with stenosis of the left anterior descending coronary artery. J Am Coll Cardiol 2005;45(8): 1186–92.

[61] Applegate R, Draughn T, Davis B. Treatment of complex LAD-diagonal bifurcation disease using paclitaxel drug-eluting stents. J Invasive Cardiol 2005;17(7):390–2.

[62] Buellesfeld L, Gerckens U, Mueller R, et al. Polymer-based paclitaxel-eluting stent for treatment of chronic total occlusions of native coronaries: Results of a Taxus CTO registry. Catheter Cardiovasc Interv 2005;66(2):173–7.

[63] Silber S, Hamburger J, Grube E, et al. Direct stenting with TAXUS stents seems to be as safe and effective as with predilatation. A post hoc analysis of TAXUS II. Herz 2004;29(2):171–80.

[64] Morice M, Colombo A, Meier B, et al. Sirolimus-vs paclitaxel-eluting stents in de novo coronary artery lesions: the REALITY trial: a randomized controlled trial. JAMA 2006;295(8):895–904.

[65] Ellis S, Popma J, Lasala J, et al. Relationship between angiographic late loss and target lesion revascularization after coronary stent implantation: analysis from the TAXUS-IV trial. J Am Coll Cardiol 2005;45(8):1193–200.

[66] Windecker S, Remondino A, Eberli F, et al. Sirolimus-eluting and paclitaxel-eluting stents for coronary revascularization. N Engl J Med 2005; 353(7):653–62.

[67] Goy J, Stauffer J, Siegenthaler M, et al. A prospective randomized comparison between paclitaxel and sirolimus stents in the real world of interventional cardiology: the TAXi trial. J Am Coll Cardiol 2005;45(2):308–11.

[68] Kastrati A, Mehilli J, von Beckerath N, et al. Sirolimus-eluting stent or paclitaxel-eluting stent vs balloon angioplasty for prevention of recurrences in patients with coronary in-stent restenosis: a randomized controlled trial. JAMA 2005;293(2):165–71.

[69] Kastrati A, Dibra A, Eberle S, et al. Sirolimus-eluting stents vs paclitaxel-eluting stents in patients with coronary artery disease: meta-analysis of randomized trials. JAMA 2005;294(7):819–25.

[70] Meredith I, Ormiston J, Whitbourn R, et al. First-in-human study of the Endeavor ABT-578-eluting phosphorylcholine-encapsulated stent system in de novo native coronary artery lesions: Endeavor I trial. Eurointervention 2005;1:157–64.

[71] Collingwood R, Gibson L, Sedlik S, et al. Stent-based delivery of ABT-578 via a phosphorylcholine surface coating reduces neointimal formation in the porcine coronary model. Catheter Cardiovasc Interv 2005;65(2):227–32.

[72] American College of Cardiology, late breaking clinical trials, March 2005.

[73] Serruys P, Sianos G, Abizaid A, et al. The effect of variable dose and release kinetics on neointimal hyperplasia using a novel paclitaxel-eluting stent platform: the Paclitaxel In-Stent Controlled Elution Study (PISCES). J Am Coll Cardiol 2005;46(2): 253–60.

[74] Tsuchida K, Piek J, Neumann FJ, et al. One-year results of a durable polymer everolimus-eluting stents in de novo coronary narrowings (The SPIRIT FIRST Trial). Eurointervention 2006, in press.

[75] Costa M, Angiolillo D, Teirstein P, et al. Sirolimus-eluting stents for treatment of complex bypass graft disease: insights from the SECURE registry. J Invasive Cardiol 2005;17(8):396–8.

[76] Serruys P, Ormiston J, Sianos G, et al. Actinomycin-eluting stent for coronary revascularization: a randomized feasibility and safety study: the ACTION trial. J Am Coll Cardiol 2004;44(7): 1363–7.

[77] Hong M, Mintz G, Lee C, et al. Paclitaxel coating reduces in-stent intimal hyperplasia in human

coronary arteries: a serial volumetric intravascular ultrasound analysis from the Asian Paclitaxel-Eluting Stent Clinical Trial (ASPECT). Circulation 2003;107(4):517–20.

[78] Park S, Shim W, Ho D, et al. A paclitaxel-eluting stent for the prevention of coronary restenosis. N Engl J Med 2003;348(16):1537–45.

[79] Gershlick A, De Scheerder I, Chevalier B, et al. Inhibition of restenosis with a paclitaxel-eluting, polymer-free coronary stent: the European evaLUation of pacliTaxel Eluting Stent (ELUTES) trial. Circulation 2004;109(4):487–93.

[80] Lansky A, Costa R, Mintz G, et al. Nonpolymer-based paclitaxel-coated coronary stents for the treatment of patients with de novo coronary lesions: angiographic follow-up of the DELIVER clinical trial. Circulation 2004;109(16):1948–54.

[81] de la Fuente L, Miano J, Mrad J, et al. Initial results of the Quanam drug-eluting stent (QuaDS-QP-2) Registry (BARDDS) in human subjects. Catheter Cardiovasc Interv 2001;53(4):480–8.

[82] Grube E, Lansky A, Hauptmann K, et al. High-dose 7-hexanoyltaxol-eluting stent with polymer sleeves for coronary revascularization: one-year results from the SCORE randomized trial. J Am Coll Cardiol 2004;44(7):1368–72.

[83] Liistro F, Stankovic G, Di MC, et al. First clinical experience with a paclitaxel derivate-eluting polymer stent system implantation for in-stent restenosis: immediate and long-term clinical and angiographic outcome. Circulation 2002;105(16):1883–6.

[84] Virmani R, Liistro F, Stankovic G, et al. Mechanism of late in-stent restenosis after implantation of a paclitaxel derivate-eluting polymer stent system in humans. Circulation 2002;106(21):2649–51.

[85] Bavry A, Kumbhani D, Helton T, et al. What is the risk of stent thrombosis associated with the use of paclitaxel-eluting stents for percutaneous coronary intervention?: a meta-analysis. J Am Coll Cardiol 2005;45(6):941–6.

[86] Ong A, Hoye A, Aoki J, et al. Thirty-day incidence and six-month clinical outcome of thrombotic stent occlusion after bare-metal, sirolimus, or paclitaxel stent implantation. J Am Coll Cardiol 2005;45(6):947–53.

[87] Katritsis D, Karvouni E, Ioannidis J. Meta-analysis comparing drug-eluting stents with bare metal stents. Am J Cardiol 2005;95(5):640–3.

[88] Jeremias A, Sylvia B, Bridges J, et al. Stent thrombosis after successful sirolimus-eluting stent implantation. Circulation 2004;109(16):1930–2.

[89] Kerner A, Gruberg L, Kapeliovich M, et al. Late stent thrombosis after implantation of a sirolimus-eluting stent. Catheter Cardiovasc Interv 2003; 60(4):505–8.

[90] Iakovou I, Schmidt T, Bonizzoni E, et al. Incidence, predictors, and outcome of thrombosis after successful implantation of drug-eluting stents. JAMA 2005;293(17):2126–30.

[91] Ong A, McFadden E, Regar E, et al. Late angiographic stent thrombosis (LAST) events with drug-eluting stents. J Am Coll Cardiol 2005; 45(12):2088–92.

[92] Kang W, Han S, Choi K, et al. Acute myocardial infarction caused by late stent thrombosis after deployment of a paclitaxel-eluting stent. J Invasive Cardiol 2005;17(7):378–80.

[93] Lee C, Tan H, Ong H, et al. Late thrombotic occlusion of paclitaxel eluting stent more than one year after stent implantation. Heart 2004;90(12):1482.

[94] Drachman D, Edelman E, Seifert P, et al. Neointimal thickening after stent delivery of paclitaxel: change in composition and arrest of growth over six months. J Am Coll Cardiol 2000;36(7):2325–32.

[95] Carter A, Aggarwal M, Kopia G, et al. Long-term effects of polymer-based, slow-release, sirolimus-eluting stents in a porcine coronary model. Cardiovasc Res 2004;63(4):617–24.

[96] Virmani R, Guagliumi G, Farb A, et al. Localized hypersensitivity and late coronary thrombosis secondary to a sirolimus-eluting stent: should we be cautious? Circulation 2004;109(6):701–5.

[97] Finn A, Kolodgie F, Harnek J, et al. Differential response of delayed healing and persistent inflammation at sites of overlapping sirolimus- or paclitaxel-eluting stents. Circulation 2005;112(2):270–8.

[98] Tanabe K, Serruys P, Degertekin M, et al. Incomplete stent apposition after implantation of paclitaxel-eluting stents or bare metal stents: insights from the randomized TAXUS II trial. Circulation 2005;111(7):900–5.

[99] Fujii K, Mintz G, Kobayashi Y, et al. Contribution of stent underexpansion to recurrence after sirolimus-eluting stent implantation for in-stent restenosis. Circulation 2004;109(9):1085–8.

[100] Kereiakes D, Kuntz R, Mauri L, et al. Surrogates, substudies, and real clinical end points in trials of drug-eluting stents. J Am Coll Cardiol 2005;45(8): 1206–12.

[101] Takebayashi H, Kobayashi Y, Dangas G, et al. Restenosis due to underexpansion of sirolimus-eluting stent in a bifurcation lesion. Catheter Cardiovasc Interv 2003;60(4):496–9.

[102] Singh H, Singh C, Aggarwal N, et al. Mycotic aneurysm of left anterior descending artery after sirolimus-eluting stent implantation: a case report. Catheter Cardiovasc Interv 2005;65(2): 282–5.

[103] Stabile E, Escolar E, Weigold G, et al. Marked malposition and aneurysm formation after sirolimus-eluting coronary stent implantation. Circulation 2004;110(5):e47–8.

[104] Vik-Mo H, Wiseth R, Hegbom K. Coronary aneurysm after implantation of a paclitaxel-eluting stent. Scand Cardiovasc J 2004;38(6):349–52.

[105] Weintraub W. Economics of sirolimus-eluting stents: drug-eluting stents have really arrived. Circulation 2004;110(5):472–4.

[106] van Hout B, Serruys P, Lemos P, et al. One-year cost-effectiveness of sirolimus-eluting stents compared with bare metal stents in the treatment of single native de novo coronary lesions: an analysis from the RAVEL trial. Heart 2005;91(4): 507–12.

[107] Cohen D, Bakhai A, Shi C, et al. Cost-effectiveness of sirolimus-eluting stents for treatment of complex coronary stenoses: results from the Sirolimus-Eluting Balloon Expandable Stent in the Treatment of Patients With De Novo Native Coronary Artery Lesions (SIRIUS) trial. Circulation 2004;110(5):508–14.

Coronary Bifurcation Lesions

Samin K. Sharma, MD, FACC*,
Annapoorna S. Kini, MD, FACC, MRCP

*Cardiac Catheterization Laboratory, Cardiovascular Institute, Mount Sinai Hospital, Box 1030,
One Gustave Levy Place, New York, NY 10029-6574, USA*

Coronary bifurcations are prone to develop atherosclerotic plaque because of turbulent blood flow and high shear stress. These lesions amount to 15% to 20% of the total number of coronary interventions. The true bifurcation lesion consists of >50% diameter obstruction of the main vessel (MV) and side branch (SB) in an inverted Y fashion.

Treatment of coronary bifurcation lesions represents a challenging area in interventional cardiology, but recent advances in percutaneous coronary interventions have led to the dramatic increase in the number of patients successfully treated percutaneously. When compared with nonbifurcation interventions, bifurcation interventions have a lower rate of procedural success, higher procedural costs, longer hospitalization, and a higher rate of clinical and angiographic restenosis [1]. The recent introduction of drug-eluting stents (DES) has resulted in a lower event rate and reduction of MV restenosis in comparison with historical controls. SB ostial residual stenosis and long-term restenosis remain a problem, however. Although stenting the MV with provisional SB stenting seems to be the prevailing approach, in the era of DES various two-stent techniques have emerged to allow stenting of the large SB (Fig. 1).

Anatomic classification

Coronary bifurcations have been classified according to the angulation between the MV

and the SB and according to the location of the plaque burden. The bifurcations are classified based on the SB angulation: (1) Y angulation: the angulation is <70° and access to the SB is usually easy, but plaque shifting is more pronounced and precise stent placement in the ostium is difficult. (2) T angulation: the angulation is >70° and access to the SB is usually more difficult, but plaque shifting is often minimal and precise stent placement in ostium is easy. Regarding plaque distribution, numerous attempts have been made to categorize bifurcations, with two classification patterns commonly used: Duke classification (Fig. 2) and Lefevre classification (Fig. 3) [2]. Although these classification patterns are used commonly, they suffer the limitations of coronary angiography (different plaque distribution and extent of disease when evaluated by intravascular ultrasound), and they do not take into account what happens to the SB on dilatation of the MV. Lesions alone in SB or MV may convert into true Y bifurcation because of plaque shift or stent protrusion during coronary intervention. Consequently, each lesion must be approached therapeutically in the context of its own anatomy and the operator's experience.

Isolated ostial lesions involving the main vessel or the side branch

With isolated ostial lesions, it is important to place a stent accurately to cover the lesion entirely without protruding into the other branch. Some operators use intravascular ultrasound to facilitate appropriate stent placement. The following techniques are suggested based on the lesion location.

---

* Corresponding author.

E-mail address: samin.sharma@msnyuhealth.org (S.K. Sharma).

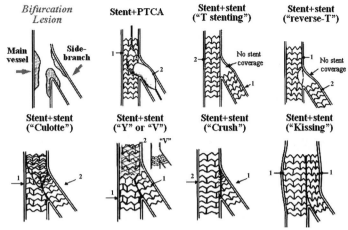

Fig. 1. Various techniques for stenting bifurcation lesions.

Isolated ostial lesion of main vessel

There are two approaches for treating these lesions: (1) placement of a stent at the ostium of the MV with a balloon protecting the SB and with inflation of the SB balloon and kissing balloon only if plaque shift occurs and (2) placement of a stent in the MV covering the origin of the SB and then wiring the SB and performing kissing balloon inflation in case the ostium of the SB deteriorates.

Isolated ostial lesions of side branch

The most common approach in treating these lesions is to place a stent at the ostium of the SB,

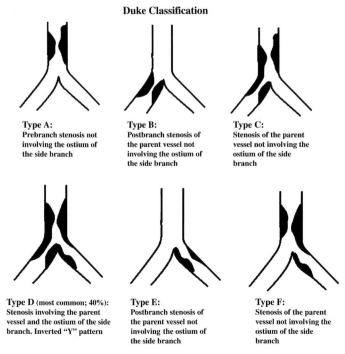

Fig. 2. Duke's classification of bifurcation lesions.

Lefevre Classification

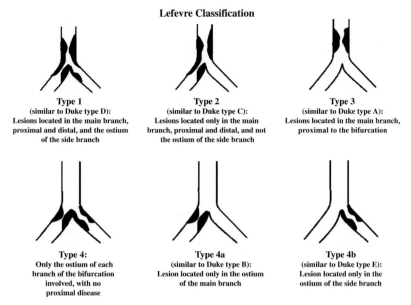

Type 1
(similar to Duke type D):
Lesions located in the main branch,
proximal and distal, and the ostium
of the side branch

Type 2
(similar to Duke type C):
Lesions located only in the main
branch, proximal and distal, and not
the ostium of the side branch

Type 3
(similar to Duke type A):
Lesions located in the main branch,
proximal to the bifurcation

Type 4:
Only the ostium of each
branch of the bifurcation
involved, with no
proximal disease

Type 4a
(similar to Duke type B):
Lesion located only in the ostium
of the main branch

Type 4b
(similar to Duke type E):
Lesion located only in the
ostium of the side branch

Fig. 3. Lefevre's classification of bifurcation lesions.

frequently with a low-pressure balloon inflated in the MV (stent pull-back technique) (Fig. 4) [3]. If after stent placement there is deterioration of the MV at the site of the bifurcation, the balloon in the MV is inflated, which protects the stent by a simultaneous inflation of the stent delivery balloon. In cases of suboptimal angiographic results in

MV, a stent can be deployed with final kissing balloon dilatation.

Impossible side branch access

There are some circumstances in which the location of the plaque in the MV or the

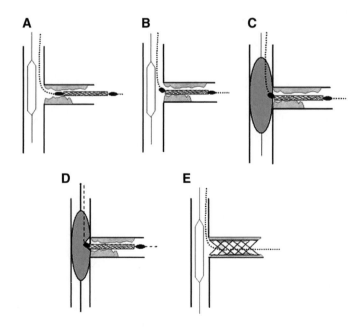

Fig. 4. Stent pull-back technique.

angulation of the SB prevents the wire from being advanced at the SB. Although rare, after attempting different types of wires with all types of curves and techniques, it still may be impossible to advance a wire in the SB. At that point few options are available: (1) Stop the procedure because the risk of losing the SB is too high, considering also the size and distribution of the branch (typically an angulated circumflex artery when stenting the distal bifurcation of an unprotected left main). (2) Perform directional coronary atherectomy on the MV with the intent of removing the plaque that prevents entry toward the SB. (3) Dilate the MV with a balloon after advancing the intended SB wire into the MV distally with the rationale that the plaque modification to a favorable plaque shift facilitates access toward the SB. After balloon dilatations, SB wire is withdrawn gently from the MV and steered gently into the SB ostium.

Selection of the guiding catheter

The selection of the size (6, 7, or 8 F) of the guiding catheter occurs after deciding whether to stent the SB. Treatment of bifurcations frequently requires simultaneous insertion of two balloons or two stents; therefore, an appropriate guiding catheter should be selected. With the currently available low-profile balloons, it is possible to insert two balloons inside a large-lumen 6-F guiding catheter with an internal lumen diameter of >0.070 in (1.75 mm). If two stents are needed, they can be inserted only one after the other, not simultaneously, in a large-lumen 6-F guiding catheter. The crush or simultaneous kissing stents technique requires a guiding catheter of minimum 7 F with an internal lumen diameter of 0.081 in (2.06 mm) or 8 F with an internal lumen diameter of 0.091 in (2.2 mm).

How many stents for the bifurcation lesion: one or two?

The strategies of using one stent (in MV) or two stents (one in MV and one in SB) for the treatment of bifurcation lesions long have been debated [4–6]. The most important initial question is whether the SB is large enough (>2.25–2.50 mm) with a sufficient territory of distribution to justify stent implantation or even balloon dilatation regardless of the bifurcation pattern. If SB is small (<1.5 mm) and supplies a small area of myocardium, it should be ignored during

percutaneous coronary intervention and a stent can be placed in the MV across the SB. There are also rare circumstances in which the SB is important and large but cannot be wired, even by expert operators using single core wires or hydrophilic wires. In these situations an operator must consider alternative options, such as coronary artery bypass surgery, if the bifurcation in question is the left main or the left anterior descending vessel and a large diagonal vessel.

The decision to use one or two stents should be made as early as possible. An appropriate and timely decision affects the results, saves time, lowers costs, and lowers the risk of complications. If the decision is made to use one stent (in the MV), the possibility almost always exists of placing a second stent on the SB in case of suboptimal results. This strategy is defined as provisional SB stenting. A recent randomized trial compared one DES (Cypher) versus two DES in the treatment of coronary bifurcation lesions [7]. This study revealed that although both techniques resulted in low angiographic restenosis of MV (approximately 5%), routine stenting of SB (two stents) was associated with a trend toward higher restenosis in the SB (23% versus 14%; $P = 0.22$) and insignificantly higher overall target lesion revascularization (TLR) (9.5% versus 4.5%; $P = 0.42$) (Fig. 5).

One stent by intention to treat: conventional (provisional) side branch stenting technique

The most common approach in the treatment of bifurcations is stenting only the MV and provisional stenting of the SB if needed for suboptimal angiographic results before or after stent deployment in the MV. The following steps are taken in this technique:

1. Wire the MV and the SB.
2. Decide the predilation device for the MV or the SB. Atherotomy devices (cutting balloon or FXminiRAIL) can be used to dilate the SB ostium with controlled focal cuts without significant dissection. Rotational atherectomy may be required in heavily calcified lesions in the MV or SB using a single bur with a bur:artery ratio of 0.4–0.5.
3. Place a stent in the MV. The stent should be deployed at a pressure of 12 to 18 atm while leaving the SB wire to prevent plaque shift, closure, or dissections in the ostium. Rarely postdilatation with a high-pressure balloon may be needed at the area of maximal plaque

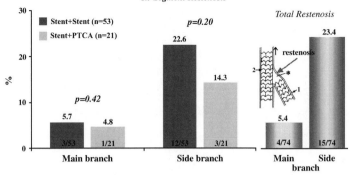

Fig. 5. The bifurcation study with Cypher Sirolimus-Eluting Stent.

burden for full stent expansion. If angiographic results in the MV and SB are satisfactory, the procedure is completed, and trapped guidewire in the SB behind the stent struts can be removed gently.

4. Place a wire into the SB to perform kissing balloon dilatations after dilatation of the SB ostium if SB ostium remained narrow or dissected. This procedure can be performed with the wire trapped behind the stent to serve as a marker. For re-entering the SB, a floppy wire, such as the Balance Universal (Guidant, Temecula, California) or Luge wire (Boston Scientific, Natick, Massachusetts), is recommended. In rare cases, a hydrophilic wire, such as the Pilot or Whisper (Guidant), cross-it (Guidant), or Asahi wire (Abbott Laboratories, Abbott Park, Illinois) is recommended. In this case, dilatation of the SB and kissing balloon inflation (usually at 8–12 atm) between the main and the SB is performed. If the result is acceptable after kissing balloon inflation, the procedure is considered complete.

5. Decide whether to stop if the result at the SB remains unsatisfactory because of difficulty in positioning a stent, size, distal runoff, or complexity of the procedure. If the decision is made to improve the result at the level of the SB, then stenting is performed according to the reverse T approach, advancing the stent via the MV stent struts with final kissing balloon dilatation.

Two stents by intention to treat

Several two-stent techniques are available, with various levels of complexity and indications:

the V, the simultaneous kissing stents, crush and its variations (reverse and step), T and its variation (modified), culottes, and Y.

The V and the simultaneous kissing stents techniques

The V technique consists of the delivery and implantation of two stents together. One stent is advanced in the SB, the other in the MV, and the two stents touch each other to form a small proximal carina (<2 mm) (Fig. 6). When the carina extends a considerable length (usually 3 mm or more) into the MV, this technique is called simultaneous kissing stents (SKS) (Fig. 7), with its modified alternative (trouser SKS) for the long lesions proximally (to avoid new long carina) (Fig. 8). The types of lesion most suitable for this technique are proximal lesions, such as distal left main bifurcation and other bifurcations with moderate to large side branch (≥2.5 mm) and vessel portion proximal to bifurcation is free of disease.

Simultaneous kissing stents technique

This technique (see Fig. 7A) involves using two appropriately sized stents (1:1 stent-to-artery ratio), one for the MV and one for the SB, with an overlap of the two stents in the proximal segment of the MV (stent sized 1:1 to the MV after the bifurcation). The proximal part of the MV should be able to accommodate the two stents, and its size should be approximately two thirds of the aggregate diameter of the two stents (eg, for two 3-mm stents in left anterior descending artery and the diagonal branch, the proximal MV size should be approximately 4 mm). Stent lengths are selected visually to cover the entire length from distal end of the SB and MV lesions to

The V Stenting Technique

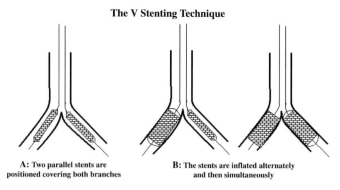

A: Two parallel stents are positioned covering both branches

B: The stents are inflated alternately and then simultaneously

Fig. 6. The V stenting technique.

proximal end in the MV. A 7- or 8-F guide catheter (internal diameter >0.78 in) is used. Debulking of MV or SB using cutting balloon or rotablator with or without balloon angioplasty is performed as clinically indicated. MV and SB are wired, and lesions with >80% stenosis are dilated by appropriate sized balloons. Two stents are advanced one by one, initially to the SB followed by one to the MV. After this step, both stents are pulled simultaneously back to the bifurcation to make a "V" and then into the proximal part of the MV to configure a "Y." The stem of the "Y" in the MV completely covers the proximal end of the lesion, with one arm of the Y in distal MV (covering the distal end of the MV lesion) and another arm in the SB (covering the distal end of SB lesions). The proximal overlapping parts of the stents are kept as short as possible but are long enough to cover the proximal end of the MV lesion.

Once the position of the stents is confirmed and proximal stent markers are overlapped, stents are deployed with simultaneous inflation at 10 to 12 atm for 10 to 20 seconds and then deflated. This procedure is followed by a second dilatation of the MV stent at 16 to 20 atm for 10 to 20 seconds to expand fully the MV stent struts while the other SB stent balloon remains deflated in the SB stent. A third dilatation of the SB stent at 14 to 20 atm for 10 to 20 seconds is performed to expand fully the SB stent struts while the other MV stent balloon remains deflated in the MV stent. This procedure is followed by the fourth and final simultaneous inflation and deflation at 10 to 12 atm for 10 to 20 seconds to form the uniform carina of the fully expanded kissing stents. Deflated stent balloons are withdrawn simultaneously. In cases of stent underexpansion, two high-pressure balloons of similar length (they

may be different size) are advanced for the simultaneous kissing balloon dilatations. In case of distal dissection, prolonged balloon dilatation is performed to avoid the need for stenting. In cases of proximal dissection, two-balloon (one in each stent) dilatation or a perfusion balloon dilatation at low pressure in the MV is performed.

Modified simultaneous kissing stents technique

In cases with a long lesion in the proximal part of MV, before bifurcation, a large stent first is deployed proximally over the guidewire in the MV (Fig. 8). It is followed by wiring the side branch via proximal stent and advancing the two stents through the MV stent to distal MV and the SB. It is deployed as described in a previous section (in a "trouser-and-seat" pattern).

During our initial experience, we compared 100 cases of SKS technique with 100 matched cases of conventional stent technique and observed lower major adverse cardica events and TLR rates in SKS versus conventional stent technique (Fig 9) [8]. Later, we analyzed our first 200 consecutive patients (202 lesions) who underwent SKS technique for true bifurcation lesions using sirolimus-eluting stents, with a minimum follow-up of 6 months (Fig. 10). Procedural success was 100% for MV and 99% for SB using SKS technique, with clinical success rate of 97%. In-hospital and 30-day major adverse cardiac events were 3% and 5%, respectively. At mean follow-up of 9 ± 2 months, the incidence of target lesion revascularization was 5% in the entire group [9].

The main advantage of these techniques is that the access to either of the two branches is never lost. When a final kissing inflation is performed, there is no need to re-cross any stent. These techniques also provide a definite SB coverage, regardless of the angulation. It is intuitive how

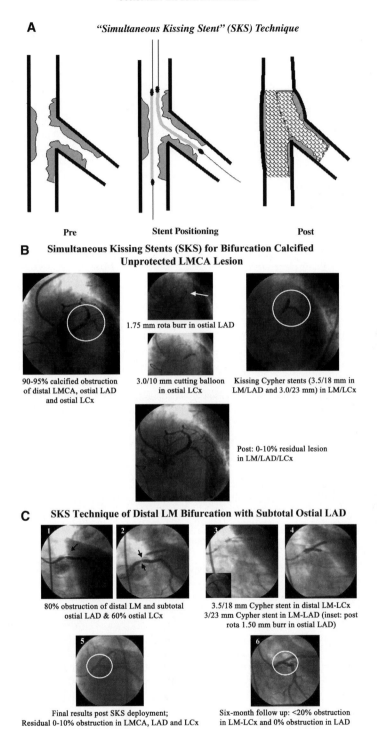

A *"Simultaneous Kissing Stent" (SKS) Technique*

Pre   Stent Positioning   Post

B Simultaneous Kissing Stents (SKS) for Bifurcation Calcified Unprotected LMCA Lesion

1.75 mm rota burr in ostial LAD

90-95% calcified obstruction of distal LMCA, ostial LAD and ostial LCx

3.0/10 mm cutting balloon in ostial LCx

Kissing Cypher stents (3.5/18 mm in LM/LAD and 3.0/23 mm) in LM/LCx

Post: 0-10% residual lesion in LM/LAD/LCx

C SKS Technique of Distal LM Bifurcation with Subtotal Ostial LAD

80% obstruction of distal LM and subtotal ostial LAD & 60% ostial LCx

3.5/18 mm Cypher stent in distal LM-LCx 3/23 mm Cypher stent in LM-LAD (inset: post rota 1.50 mm burr in ostial LAD)

Final results post SKS deployment; Residual 0-10% obstruction in LMCA, LAD and LCx

Six-month follow up: <20% obstruction in LM-LCx and 0% obstruction in LAD

Fig. 7. (*A*) The SKS technique. (*B*) SKS technique for bifurcation calcified unprotected left main coronary artery lesion. (*C*) SKS technique of distal left main bifurcation with subtotal ostial left anterior descending.

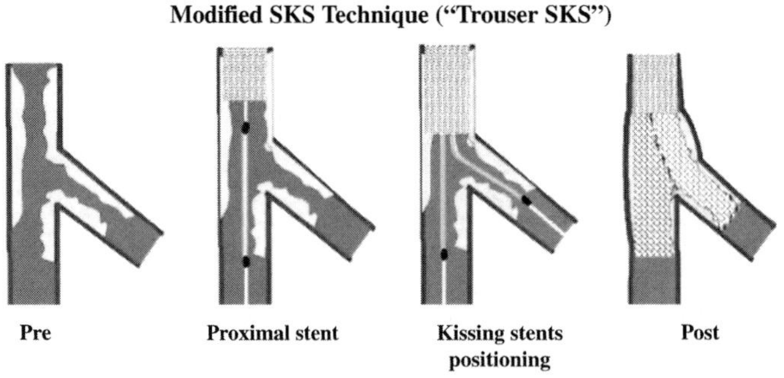

Modified SKS Technique ("Trouser SKS")

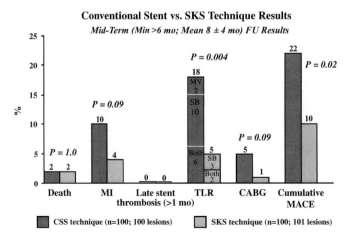

| Pre | Proximal stent | Kissing stents positioning | Post |

Fig. 8. The modified SKS (trouser SKS) technique (for long lesions).

problematic the need may be to position a stent proximal to the double barrel. There is an inevitable bias toward one of the two branches and the high likelihood of leaving a gap. If there is a need to place a stent at the proximal segment of a vessel treated with SKS stenting, two options are available: (1) a stent is placed proximally, which leaves a small gap between the kissing stents and the proximal stent and (2) the kissing stent technique is converted into a crush technique, with the stent in the MV compressing the other stent (one arm of the V) in the SB. A wire crosses the struts into the SB, and a balloon is inflated toward the SB. After wire removal from the SB, the proximal stent is advanced toward the MV.

The crush technique

The crush technique was introduced at the time of DES introduction and is described schematically in Fig. 11. Two stents are placed in the MV and the SB, with the former more proximal than the latter. The stent of the SB is deployed, and its balloon and wire are removed. The stent subsequently deployed in the MV flattens the protruding cells of the SB stent—hence the name crushing or crush technique. Wire re-crossing and dilatation of the SB with a balloon of a diameter at least equal to that of the stent and then final kissing balloon inflation are recommended. The implementation of final kissing balloon inflation is performed to allow better strut contact against the ostium of the SB and better drug delivery. Follow-up studies have shown that if restenosis occurs, this narrowing is focal (<5 mm in length) and most of the time is not associated with symptoms or ischemia [10].

Ge and colleagues [11] published a study to evaluate the long-term outcomes after implantation of DES in bifurcation lesions with the crush technique. Although the long-term outcome of crush stenting technique has yet to be determined, results of this study showed that compared with

Fig. 9. SKS versus conventional stent technique: follow-up results.

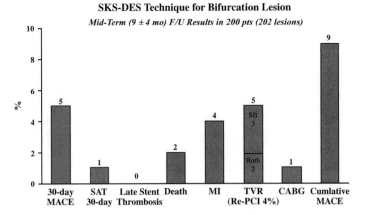

Fig. 10. SKS-DES technique for bifurcation lesions.

the absence of kissing balloon after dilation, the crush stenting with kissing balloon after dilation seems to be associated with more favorable long-term outcomes (Fig. 12). When using the crush stenting technique, kissing balloon after dilation is mandatory to reduce the restenosis rate of SB and the need for TLR.

The main advantage of the crush technique is that the immediate patency of both branches is assured. This technique also provides excellent

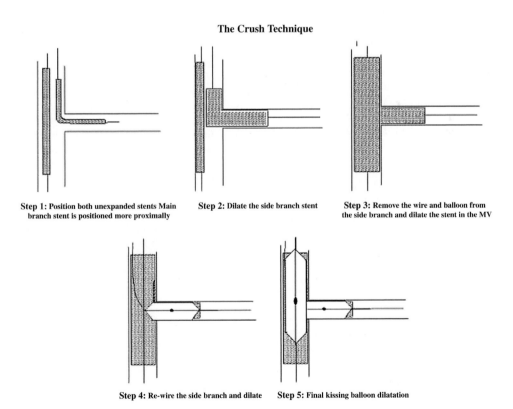

Fig. 11. The crush technique.

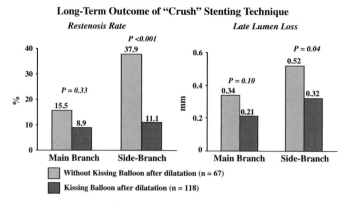

Fig. 12. Long-term outcome of crush stenting technique.

coverage of the ostium of the SB. The main disadvantage is that the performance of the final kissing balloon inflation makes the procedure more laborious because of the need to re-cross multiple struts with a wire and balloon.

The reverse crush

The main indication for performing the reverse crush is to allow an opportunity for provisional SB stenting. A stent is deployed in the MV, and balloon dilatation with final kissing inflation toward the SB is performed. It is assumed that the result of the SB is suboptimal and stent placement will be needed. A second stent is advanced into the SB and left in position without being deployed. A balloon sized according to the diameter of the MV is positioned at the level of the bifurcation, and the surgeon ensures that it stays inside the previously deployed MV stent. The stent in the SB is retracted approximately 2 to 3 mm into the MV and deployed, the deploying balloon is removed, and an angiogram is obtained to verify that a good result is present at the SB (no further distal stent in the SB is needed). If this is the case, the wire from the SB is removed and the balloon in the MV is inflated at high pressure, with final steps involving re-crossing into the SB, performing SB dilatation, and final kissing balloon inflation.

The main advantages of the reverse crush technique are that the immediate patency of both branches is assured and the technique can be performed using a 6-F guiding catheter. This technique has the same disadvantages as the standard crush but is more laborious.

T technique

The classic T technique consists of positioning a stent first at the ostium of the SB while being

careful to avoid stent protrusion into the MV (Fig. 13). Some operators leave a balloon in the MV to help to further locate the MV. After deployment of the stent and removal of the balloon and the wire from the SB, a second stent is advanced in the MV. A wire is then re-advanced into the SB, and final kissing balloon inflation is performed. Modified T stenting is a variation performed by simultaneously positioning stents at the SB and the MV [12]. The SB stent is deployed first, and after wire and balloon removal from the SB, the MV stent is deployed. The reverse T stenting technique is used when SB ostium deteriorates after stent deployment in the MV, which requires re-crossing the SB, dilating, and then advancing the stent in the SB. A final kissing balloon dilatation is recommended.

This technique is simple and technically less demanding. It can be used for the coverage of lesions located proximal to the bifurcation. In almost all cases, this technique leads to incomplete coverage of the ostium of the SB.

The culottes technique

The culottes technique uses two stents and leads to full coverage of the bifurcation at the expense of an excess of metal covering of the proximal end (Fig. 14). Both branches are predilated. First a stent is deployed across the most angulated branch, usually the SB. The nonstented branch is then rewired through the struts of the stent and dilated. A second stent is advanced and expanded into the nonstented branch, usually the MV. Finally, kissing balloon inflation is performed [13].

This technique is suitable for all angles of bifurcations and provides near-perfect coverage of the SB ostium. This technique also leads to a high

The T Stenting Technique

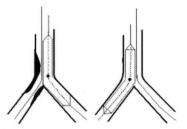

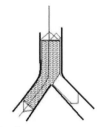

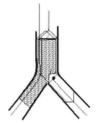

Step 1: Wire both branches and dilate alternatively or simultaneously the main and the side branch

Step 2: Remove wire from the side branch and stent the main branch

Step 3: Maintain the wire in the main branch. With a second wire, cross the stent into the unstented vessel and dilate the stent

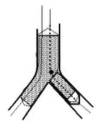

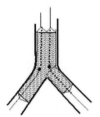

Step 4: Implant a second stent at the ostium of the side branch; can be performed before stenting the main branch (avoids difficulties of stenting through a stent, increases risk in case of incorrect positioning)

Step 5: Perform final kissing balloon dilatation

Fig. 13. The T stenting technique.

concentration of metal with a double-stent layer at the carina and in the proximal part of the bifurcation. The main disadvantage of the technique is that rewiring both branches through the stent struts can be difficult and time consuming.

The Y technique

This technique involves an initial predilatation followed by stent deployment in each branch (Fig. 15). If the results are not adequate, a third stent may be deployed in the MV. Currently this technique is not commonly used.

This technique is a last resort for treating demanding bifurcations in which there is a need to maintain wire access to both branches. The major limitations of this approach are the need to modify the delivery system of the proximal stent and manually crimp the stent on two balloons, which could be problematic with DES.

Lesion preparation before proceeding with the intervention

Plaque removal before stent implantation using directional atherectomy in noncalcified lesions

and rotational atherectomy in calcified lesions has been attractive. Some encouraging results of many single-center experiences have not been reproduced in the randomized trials, however. Rotational atherectomy in the heavily calcified lesions is the only procedure to permit adequate lesion dilatation and subsequent stent delivery. Early reports stated an advantage in facilitating stent delivery and expansion, with a suggestion for clinical benefit when used in calcified lesions. The Stenting Post Rotational Atherectomy (SPORT) randomized study, which used rotational atherectomy and stenting, failed to support any advantage of this technology over standard bare metal stenting. Most of the time, rotablation is performed only on the MV, but occasionally also or only on the SB. We think that especially with the use of DES, lesion preparation with compliance change for a calcified lesion can facilitate stent delivery and symmetrical stent expansion substantially with more homogeneous drug delivery. Several single-center studies reported the beneficial combination of stenting preceded by cutting balloon dilatation. In bifurcation lesions, in which a large fibrotic plaque

The Culottes Stenting Technique

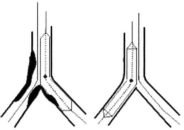

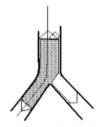

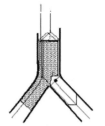

Step 1: Both branches are wired and dilated   Step 2: Remove wire from the straighter branch and deploy the stent in the more angulated branch   Step 3: Remove the wire from the other branch

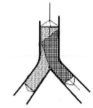

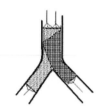

Step 4: Position the second stent towards the unstented second branch and expand the stent leaving proximal overlap   Step 5: Recross the first stent with the wire and perform final kissing balloon inflation.

Fig. 14. The culottes stenting technique.

is present at the ostium of the SB, the use of the cutting balloon as a predilatation strategy before stenting seems reasonable.

Currently, we suggest the use of the cutting balloon in moderately calcific and fibrotic lesions, especially ones that involve the origin of the SB. In heavily calcified lesions, instead of using a larger bur, the cutting balloon could be used after small-bur rotablation with the goal of minimizing any distal embolization. Symmetric stent expansion, avoidance of SB recoil, and stent compression are all attractive hypotheses that need proper evaluation.

Adjunct pharmacotherapy

Preprocedural heparin administration in doses of 100 U/kg without and 70 U/kg with glycoprotein IIb/IIIa inhibitors to keep activated clotting time between 250 and 300 sec is recommended. Use of glycoprotein IIb/IIIa inhibitors is encouraged, especially in patients who have thrombus-containing lesions or acute coronary syndromes, with use of rotational atherectomy, and for use with multiple long stents. These agents are sometimes administered when the final result at the SB seems suboptimal and the operator wishes to

avoid implanting another stent. Periprocedural preparation with thienopyridines with a 600-mg loading dose of clopidogrel is routinely used. The duration of combined thienopyridine and aspirin treatment after stent implantation should be emphasized strictly for a minimum of 1 year, with extended duration in severely complex cases using multiple stents to avoid delayed stent thrombosis [14].

Future directions and summary

Based on the size of the SB, an algorithm can be created in the treatment of bifurcation lesions. As a conclusion, Fig. 16 shows a suggested algorithm for treatment of bifurcation coronary lesions. A wire should be placed in the SB, especially if there is disease at the ostium or there is a problematic takeoff. The general consensus is to try to keep the procedure safe and simple. When the SB is not severely diseased, implantation of a stent in the MV and provisional stenting in the SB is the preferred strategy. Implantation of two stents as the initial approach is appropriate when both branches are significantly diseased and SB is >2.5 mm. Final kissing balloon inflation should be performed in these cases.

The Y Stenting Technique

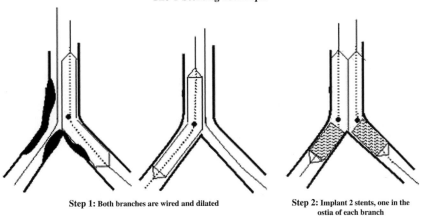

Step 1: Both branches are wired and dilated

Step 2: Implant 2 stents, one in the ostia of each branch

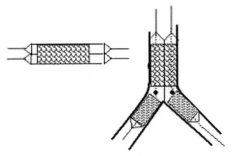

Step 3: A proximal stent is crimped on two balloons, advanced to the carina and deployed by inflating both balloons simultaneously; Alternatively, the proximal stent can be mounted on one balloon followed by final kissing balloon inflation.

Fig. 15. The Y stenting technique.

The ongoing randomized trials entitled "Coronary bifurcations: Application of the Crushing Technique Using Sirolimus-eluting stents" (CACTUS), which compare a provisional SB strategy with the crush technique using Cypher stents, and a pilot trial for treatment of true bifurcation lesions with simultaneous kissing stents (Precise-SKS trial) may help to answer better the approach of one versus two stents in true bifurcation lesions. Although dedicated stents are being developed (ie, petal stent [Boston Scientific Corp.], which has a side hole covered by a 2-mm metal

Interventional Algorithm for Bifurcation Lesions

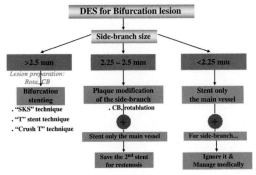

Fig. 16. Interventional algorithm for bifurcation lesions.

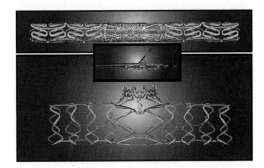

Fig. 17. Petal stent.

protrusion [Fig. 17]), their clinical use in the format of DES is still limited. These devices potentially may have important applications in proximal large bifurcations and in the left main trunk.

In summary, major achievements in the stenting of bifurcation lesions since the introduction of DES are single-digit restenosis rates on the MV and focal restenosis at the SB, which is frequently clinically silent [15,16].

References

[1] Dauerman H, Higgins P, Sparano A, et al. Mechanical debulking versus balloon angioplasty for the treatment of true bifurcation lesions. J Am Coll Cardiol 1998;32:1845–52.

[2] Lefevre T, Louvard Y, Morice MC, et al. Stenting of bifurcation lesions: classification, treatments, and results. Catheter Cardiovasc Interv 2000;49:274–83.

[3] Kini A, Moreno P, Steinheimer A, et al. Effectiveness of the stent pull-back technique for non-aorto ostial coronary narrowings. Am J Cardiol 2005;96: 1123–8.

[4] Al Suwaidi J, Berger P, Rihal C, et al. Immediate and long-term outcome of intracoronary stent implantation for true bifurcation lesions. J Am Coll Cardiol 2000;35:929–36.

[5] Yamashita T, Nishida T, Adamian M, et al. Bifurcation lesions: two stents versus one stent. Immediate and follow-up results. J Am Coll Cardiol 2000;35: 1145–51.

[6] Pan M, de Lezo SJ, Medina A, et al. Simple and complex stent strategies for bifurcated coronary arterial stenosis involving the side-branch origin. Am J Cardiol 1999;83:1320–5.

[7] Colombo A, Moses J, Morice M, et al. Randomized study to evaluate sirolimus-eluting stents implanted at coronary bifurcation lesions. Circulation 2004; 109:1244–9.

[8] Sharma S, Ahsan C, Lee J, et al. Simultaneous kissing stents (SKS) technique for treating bifurcation lesions in medium-to-large size coronary arteries. Am J Cardiol 2004;94:913–7.

[9] Sharma SK. Simultaneous kissing drug-eluting stent technique for percutaneous treatment of bifurcation lesions in large-size vessels. Catheter Cardiovasc Interv 2005;65:10–6.

[10] Colombo A, Stankovic G, Orlic D, et al. Modified T-stenting technique with crushing for bifurcation lesions: immediate results and 30-day outcome. Catheter Cardiovasc Interv 2003;60:145–51.

[11] Ge L, Airoldi F, Iakovou I, et al. Clinical and angiographic outcome after implantation of drug-eluting stents in bifurcation lesions with the crush stent technique: importance of final kissing balloon postdilation. J Am Coll Cardiol 2005;46:613–20.

[12] Kobayashi Y, Colombo A, Akiyama T, et al. Modified "T" stenting: a technique for kissing stents in bifurcational coronary lesions. Cathet Cardiovasc Diagn 1998;43:323–6.

[13] Chevalier B, Glatt B, Royer T, et al. Placement of coronary stents in bifurcation lesions by the "culotte" technique. Am J Cardiol 1998;82:943–9.

[14] Iakovou I, Schmidt T, Bonizzoni E, et al. Incidence, prediction and outcome of thrombosis after successful implantation of drug-eluting stents. JAMA 2005; 293:2126–30.

[15] Pan M, de Lezo SJ, Medina A, et al. Rapamycin-eluting stents for the treatment of bifurcated coronary lesions; a randomized comparison of a simple versus complex strategy. Am Heart J 2004;148: 857–64.

[16] Toutouzas K, Stankovic G, Takagi T, et al. A new dedicated stent and delivery system for the treatment of bifurcation lesions: preliminary experience. Catheter Cardiovasc Interv 2003;58:34–42.

Chronic Total Coronary Occlusions

Gregory A. Braden, MD

Cardiology Specialists of North Carolina, 3866 Cedarfield Place Court, Winston-Salem, NC 27106, USA

Chronic total coronary occlusions (CTOs) occur in up to one third of patients undergoing coronary angiography and have become the final frontier of interventional cardiology. Anatomically, CTOs typically consist of a hard fibrocalcific proximal cap, a distal cap with generally less fibrotic material, and a central area of organized thrombus. Indications for opening CTOs include relief of angina, improved left ventricular function, and improved long-term survival. The fibro-calcific nature of these occlusions is responsible for the somewhat lower success rates in opening these lesions, predominantly by increasing the difficulty in passing the occlusion with a guidewire. Newer technology, wire-based and non–wire-based, has improved the ability to cross these previously uncrossable lesions, thereby improving the acute success rates of opening these lesions. Stenting improved long-term patency rates for these lesions, and now drug-eluting stents have made the late restenosis rates similar to those seen for nonoccluded arteries. Therefore, the clinical imperative for opening these arteries has increased.

CTOs are defined as occlusions in the coronary arteries with Thrombolysis in Myocardial Infarction (TIMI) 0 flow or functional occlusions with TIMI 1 flow (penetration of contrast without filling of the distal vessel) of at least 1-month duration. Age criteria in various studies have ranged from 2 weeks to 3 months but are difficult to assess unless serial angiograms are available. Thus age often is difficult to define and is dependent on clinical history [1–4]. A prior history of myocardial infarction (MI) was present in 42% to 68% of patients who had angiographically documented CTOs [5–9]. The prevalence of CTOs is high, occurring in approximately one third of patients undergoing coronary angiography [10]. Not surprisingly, the incidence of CTOs seems to increase with patient age, especially in the left anterior descending coronary artery (LAD) distribution [11]. The presence of one or more CTOs was an angiographic exclusion for randomization in 43% of patients ineligible for the German Angioplasty Bypass Investigation [12] and for 35% of patients who had angiographic exclusions for the Balloon Angioplasty Revascularization Investigation (BARI) trials [13]. Accordingly, although CTOs represented 30% to 40% of patients listed in the National Cardiovascular Registry of the American Collage of Cardiology, CTO angioplasty accounted for only 12% of procedures between January 1998 and September 2000 in 139 United States hospitals [14].

Clinical indications for treating chronic total coronary occlusions

The rationale for treating CTOs follows several lines of evidence; the strongest include improved survival with successful procedures. The Mid-America Heart Institute published the results of a 10-year retrospective analysis of 2007 patients who had CTOs in whom percutaneous coronary intervention (PCI) was attempted and matched those patients with 2007 patients undergoing PCI for nonocclusive disease between 1980 and 1999. There was a 74.4% success rate in the CTO group. Better in-hospital outcomes were associated with a successful procedure (major adverse coronary event [MACE] rate of 3.2% versus 5.4%; $P = .02$). Similarly, there was an improved 10-year survival advantage associated with a successful procedure (successful 73.5% versus unsuccessful 65.0%; $P = .001$). The long-term outcome of

E-mail address: GBraden@triad.rr.com

CTOs successfully recanalized was similar to successful procedures in the matched cohort of patients undergoing PCI for nonocclusive disease (73.5% versus 71.9%; P = not significant) [15]. Several other registries have shown similar results. There was a 56% (P < .001) reduction in relative risk for mortality over 7 years' follow-up in the British Columbia Cardiac Registry in which 1458 patients who had CTO were treated [16]. The Total Occlusion Angioplasty Study-Societa Italiana di Cardiologia Invasiva (TOAST-GISE) showed a similar result in a smaller cohort of patients (369 patients) over a shorter follow-up (1 year), with a reduced incidence of cardiac death or MI with successful procedures (1.1% versus 6.2%; P = .005) [15]. In the only study incorporating stent use to a significant degree, the Thorax Center reported 5-year follow-up of 885 consecutive patients who had CTO treated from 1992 through 2002. There was a 65.1% success rate in these patients. Successful procedures were again associated with improved 5-year survival (93.5% versus 88.0%; P = .02) [17].

Besides a survival benefit seen from of treating CTOs, improvements in clinical symptoms, improvements in left ventricular function, and a reduced need for late coronary bypass surgery (CABG) have been associated with successful opening of CTOs. There was a greater freedom from angina in TOAST-GISE for successful procedures (88.7% versus 75.0%; P = .008) [5]. Left ventricular function improved in a series of 95 patients studied at baseline and at 6.7 ± 1.4 months. Left ventricular ejection fraction increased from $625 \pm 13\%$ to $675 \pm 11\%$ (P < .001) with opening these occluded arteries [18,19]. Chung and colleagues [20] showed a similar effect in a population of 75 patients who did not have known MI, demonstrating an improvement in ejection fraction from 59.5% to 67.3% (P < .001), but not in a similar group with a previously documented MI (48.9% to 50.5%; P = not significant). Finally, TOAST-GISE showed a decreased need for late CABG in patients who had successful PCI of CTOs (2.5% versus 15.7%; P < .001) [5]. The presence of a CTO was the major angiographic exclusion for both the BARI [20] and Emory Angioplasty versus Surgery Trials [5].

Histopathology of chronic total coronary occlusions

Insight into the difficulty of opening CTOs and their propensity for complications and restenosis can be understood better by examining the histopathology of CTOs. CTOs generally occur after thrombotic occlusion of the coronary artery as a result of a ruptured plaque. The thrombus organizes as it ages, with various amounts of calcification, fibrosis, and inflammation. Generally, there is more fibro-calcific plaque at the proximal cap and at the distal cap. Often the middle section remains soft, with organized thrombus present. There is a variable amount of neovascularization present. Neovascularization seems to be an early event. Occasionally, the channels can become large and influence guidewire passage. The amount of calcification is somewhat related to the age of the CTO, although there can be extensive calcification even in younger occlusions (<3 months). The amount of calcification may predict the ability to cross the total occlusion with a guidewire and may cause the guidewire to deflect behind the plaque into the subintimal space during an attempt to cross [21,22]. CTO vessels may undergo a significant amount of negative remodeling, probably secondary to a chronic decrease in perfusion pressure or to adventitial responses to neovascularization [23].

Patient selection

Certain angiographic and clinical features have been associated with higher success rates for opening totally occluded coronary arteries. Angiographic features include the presence of a tapered stump at the occlusion site and the presence of microchannels (subtotally occluded arteries). The features that have been associated with a lower likelihood of success include the presence of a blunt or flush occlusion, the presence of the occlusion at a side branch, small vessel size, marked tortuosity, and heavy calcification. The presence of bridging collaterals also negatively impacts outcome with CTOs. Lesion length also predictably affects outcomes, with longer occlusions having worse results and short occlusions better chance of success. Nonvisualization of the distal bed remains a strong contraindication to attempting CTOs using percutaneous techniques. Clinically, the duration of occlusion has been associated with success, so that long-duration occlusions are more difficult to cross. The development of newer CTO specialty guidewires and newer nonguidewire technology has made some of the negative predictors of success obsolete.

Procedural techniques for chronic total coronary occlusions

Like many complex catheterization laboratory procedures, CTO interventional outcomes are highly technique dependant. Patient selection, equipment selection, and procedure conduct all affect outcomes.

Equipment selection for CTOs involves the selection of guide catheters, support catheters, guidewires, and new-generation technology for crossing these lesions as well as the final dilatation strategies once across (Figs. 1 and 2).

Guide catheters should be chosen to provide both good back-up support and good coaxial alignment with the coronary ostium. For the left system, curved shapes such as extra backup or extra support are best, but occasionally, an Amplatz shape for the circumflex provides the best support. In the right system, backup support is dependent on the orientation of the right coronary artery (RCA) along with its course after the take-off. In general, curves such as a hockey-stick shape provide moderate support, and a right or left Amplatz provides more aggressive support, but these shapes have a tendency to deep seat the coronary artery and therefore have more chance

of dissecting the proximal RCA or the aorta. Although there has been a migration toward the use of smaller guide catheters, the CTO angioplasty generally is preformed better with larger-lumen guides such as 7 or 8 Fr. The larger-caliber guides give better backup support and allow the use of multiple guidewires and balloon or support catheters.

Guidewire technology has evolved rather rapidly. The ideal guidewire would provide nearly one-to-one torque response with the ability to shape the tip in infinite configurations and to retain the tip shape with use. Additionally, the tip should be atraumatic but should have enough stiffness to penetrate the hard fibro-calcific caps. The frictional losses in feel along the guidewire should be such that the feel of the tip is maintained despite proximal tortuosity and calcification. Unfortunately, the ideal guidewire does not exist. Previously, soft-tipped or intermediate guidewires were the initial choice for attempting to open CTOs. In the mid 1990s specialty CTO guidewires with tapered tips were developed to address issues with standard guidewires. This development paralleled the development of hydrophilic guidewires for coronary use and led to a debate concerning the use of hydrophilic versus

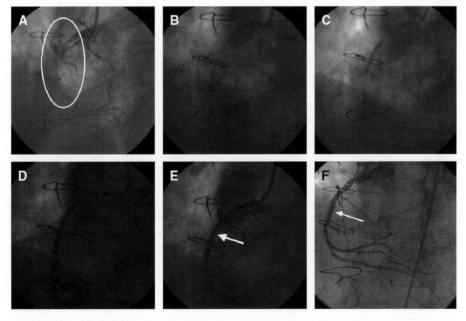

Fig. 1. Rota plus drug-eluting stent (Taxus) of CTO (12 years old) of RCA with 12-month follow-up. (*A*) Long total occlusion of RCA with bridge collaterals (*within white oval*). (*B,C*) 1.25 mm Rota burr and 2.5/20 mm Maverick II balloon (Boston Scientific, Maplegrove, MN). (*D*) 3.5/32.0 mm Taxus stent in RCS. (*E*) 0–10% residual obstruction (*arrow*). (*F*) No angiographic or clinical restenosis is seen at 1-year follow-up (*arrow*).

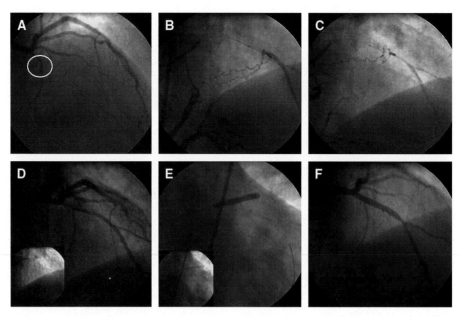

Fig. 2. CTO of the LAD: Safe-Cross RF wire followed by Rota plus drug-eluting stent (Cypher, Cordis Corp., Miami Lakes, FL). (*A*) 100% long calcified lesion of mid-LAD with bridge collaterals (*within white circle*). (*B*) 0.010 inch Cross It 300 wire (Guidant) in false lumen as shown in the contralateral RCA injection. (*C*) Safe-Cross RF wire advance in the true lumen after seen bursts of RF energy. (*D*) After Rota plus percutaneous transluminal coronary angioplasty using 3.0/20 mm Maverick balloon at 6 atmospheres (1.25 mm Rota burr ablation for 55 seconds at 142,000 rpm). (*E*) 3.5/33 mm Cypher stent in proximal LAD. (*F*) After drug-eluting stent: 0–10% residual lesion in proximal mid-LAD.

hydrophobic guidewires for crossing CTOs. Hydrophilic guidewires generally are used for crossing lesions that are subtotally occluded, with the possibility that the hydrophilic wire might find microchannels and traverse the CTO more easily. Additionally, if there is marked tortuosity and calcification proximally, there may be a benefit in using hydrophilic wires to decrease the friction and improve the manipulation of the wire. Otherwise, most operators prefer hydrophobic anode wires to optimize the feel of the lesion. Recently unibody, solid-core wires with excellent tip-shaping properties have been developed in Japan by Asahi Intec and marketed in the United States by Abbott Vascular (Redwood City, California). These devices include both the Miraclebros and Confienza lines. These two wire lines are similar in construction, except that the Confienza is tapered to 0.01 inches at the tip. The Confienza is also available as a hybrid wire (Confienza Pro), which has a hydrophilic coating except for the distal 5 mm of the tip. The Miraclebros series come in various tip stiffness from 3 to 12 g force, whereas the Confienza has a 9-g tip. These wires have improved the crossability of CTOs. Medtronic (Santa Rosa, California) has recently introduced

a similar line of CTO wires called the Predator series. Guidant (Tamacula, California) has introduced a CTO subspecialty wire of 0.010 inches of various stiffness (100–400x) with a nonhydrophilic stiff tip to facilitate the penetration of fibrous cap but minimize the subintimal passage of the wire. In general, one would start with a softer-tipped, less traumatic guidewire and advance in stiffness to penetrate the CTO while minimizing the risk of dissection/perforation.

Support catheters are important in treating CTOs for various reasons. Support catheters provide the ability to exchange guidewires easily or to change the shape of the wire tip during use. Additionally, the use of a support catheter decreases the friction associated with wire placement and manipulation and provides additional backup for the wire to penetrate tough lesions. Various types of support catheters are available, including low-profile, over-the-wire balloons, generally 1.5- or 2.0-mm short balloons. Selective infusion catheters similar to the Transit Catheter (Cordis, Miami, Florida), the Spectronetics (Westbury, New York) Quick-Cross support catheter, the Intraluminal (Carlsbad, California) Therapeutics angled support catheter, and St Jude's

(St. Paul, Minnesota) Venture catheter, which allows different tip deflections in vivo, thus providing different angles to the catheter. The Tornus catheter (Abbott Vascular) is both a support catheter and penetration catheter for uncrossable lesions.

The planning and conduct of the approach for opening CTOs is important. To determine the path of the vessel in the CTO segment, it is necessary to take angiograms in multiple projections. The use of biplanar angiography saves time and provides an easier method for obtaining multiple angiographic projections. It is important to define the distal vascular bed beyond the CTO. Sometimes there are adequate homo-collaterals for the distal vessel to be seen well. More often, however, it is necessary to inject the contralateral vessel to define the vessel distal, using collaterals to see beyond the CTO well. The ability to see this distal vessel is one of the most important steps to wiring the CTO successfully.

During guidewire manipulation the guidewire may end up in a blind pouch behind the plaque associated with the CTO. If this occurs, it is very difficult to recross the plaque and re-enter the true lumen. In this situation, if the current guidewire is left in place and a second guidewire is introduced, the first guidewire serves as a landmark for the false channel created and may prevent (block) the second guidewire form entering this false channel. This technique has been termed the "see-saw" or "parallel-wire" technique.

Another technique described by Antonio Colombo and colleagues [24] uses a subintimal path predominantly in the RCA. A 0.014-inch hydrophilic guide with a J configuration is purposely advanced in the subintimal space beyond the CTO, and re-entry into the true lumen is attempted in the distal vessel using a guidewire with a sharply bent tip. This technique has been termed the "subintimal tracking and re-entry" (STAR) technique. This technique should be attempted only in the RCA, where the risk of occluding major side branches is minimized.

Nonguidewire novel devices for chronic total coronary occlusions

Newer, nonguidewire approaches for the treatment of CTOs have been approved. These include the Intraluminal Therapeutics (ILT) Safe-Cross and the LuMend (Red Wood City, California) Frontrunner catheters. The Safe-Cross system uses a 0.014-inch guidewire sleeve, which incorporates a fiberoptic wire and transmission wire to image and to deliver radio-frequency (RF) energy for the ablation of plaque. The imaging is forward looking with a resolution of 100 μ, providing a signal to determine the proximity of the tip of the guidewire to the vessel wall. It then can deliver RF energy to the catheter tip to ablate plaque, including calcified plaque. Using the imaging array to avoid the outer vessel, the wire can be redirected through the true lumen if progress is not being made in crossing the CTO. Using RF energy when necessary, the wire can be navigated across the CTO while incorporating the imaging. The value of the Safe-Cross system was seen in the Guided Radio Frequency Energy Ablation of Total Occlusions registry where Safe-Cross system was used after an attempt with a conventional guidewire for at least 10 minutes of flouro-time failed to cross the lesion. In the trial, there was a 54.3% success rate in these conventional guidewire failures. These device has a significant learning curve, because there was a marked difference in the success rate between the first half and the second half of the study (41.6% versus 67%; $P <$ .01) [25]. There are also 0.018-inch and 0.035-inch Safe-Cross guidewires for the use in the periphery.

The other new device receiving Food and Drug Administration approval for use in CTOs is the Lumend Frontrunner catheter. This catheter uses blunt dissection to negotiate through CTOs. Jaws at the tip of the catheter open and close to push plaque aside to go through or around the plaque and make a channel through the CTO. Once across, the frontrunner catheter is replaced with a guidewire beyond the CTO, and the lesion is treated with balloon angioplasty or stenting. A registry trial was preformed for approval in guidewire-refractory lesions using 10 minutes of flouro-time. The Frontrunner was successful in reaching the distal lumen in 56.1% of these guidewire-refractory cases [26]. Severe acute complications with both of these devices were low and occurred in less than 1% of cases.

There are other devices under study in an attempt to increase success rates for CTOs or to decrease the time required with its antecedent use of contrast and radiography to treat CTOs. Closest to market is the FlowCardia (FlowCardia, Inc., Sunnyvale, California). Crosser system using vibrational energy transmitted down a catheter to jackhammer open the CTO [27]. The Crosser uses a nitinol wire, which has low energy losses, as the transmission wire. Initial results demonstrate a 64.2% success rate for guidewire-refractory lesions with an excellent safety profile. Other devices are in the design and early feasibility stages of development [28].

Outcomes of chronic total coronary occlusions

The short- and long-term outcomes of CTO intervention have been variable over time and with operator experience. CTO intervention represents between 6% and 10% of the total PCIs preformed in the United States, thus representing nearly 100,000 procedures annually. Therefore, the outcome of this patient population contributes in a significant way to total PCI outcome in the United States.

The acute success rate for opening CTOs has increased in contemporary series because of improved technology, a better understanding of the pathobiology of CTOs, and operator experience with improved techniques. Generally, published series have an acute success rate of 50% to 80%, but the reported success rate may be an overestimation resulting from a selection bias in the data submitted for publication. In any circumstance, this patient population clearly has the lowest acute success rate and probably represents the last frontier to impact angioplasty results dramatically. The most common mode of failure in unsuccessful cases included failure to cross with a guidewire (in approximately 80% to 90% of cases), failure to cross with a balloon (in approximately 10% to 15% of cases), and failure to dilate a resistant lesion (in the remaining approximately 2% to 5% of cases). Strategies incorporating stiffer guidewires, more backup support from guide catheters and support catheters, and newer non–wire-based technologies are addressing these issues. The inability to cross with a balloon is addressed typically by changing to a Rotablator wire (Boston Scientific, Maple Grove, Minnesota) and treating the lesion with the excimer laser (Spectronetics) over the wire that crossed the CTO. Recently, the Tornus catheter (Abbott Vascular) has been used as both a wire-support catheter and as a drilling-type catheter to cross some resistant lesions.

Long-term success rates traditionally have been less than ideal, with high restenosis rates and high reocclusion rates compared with PCI of nonoccluded vessels. Various randomized trials comparing percutaneous transluminal coronary angioplasty with stenting with bare metal stents have provided insight into these long-term outcomes. Restenosis rates for balloon angioplasty of CTOs have ranged from 33% to 74%. Additionally, the reocclusion rates have been high, ranging

from 7% to 34% in various studies. The use of stents has improved these outcomes markedly. With bare metal stents, the restenosis rates have declined by approximately 40%, ranging from 22% to 55% [5,9]. Likewise, late reocclusion rates have declined with stenting by more than 50%, ranging from 2% to 16%. With the advent of drug-eluting stents, these restenosis rates have improved. Although no randomized trials have been completed, insight into the effect of drug-eluting stents on restenosis can be gleaned from several registries. In the Rapamycin-Eluting Stent evaluated at Rotterdam Cardiology Hospital registry from the Thorax Center in Rotterdam, The Netherlands, the 1-year event-free survival for CTOs treated with sirolimus-eluting stents was 96.4%, compared with a 82.8% event-free survival rate in a matched, consecutive series of patients treated with bare metal stents [29]. In a series of 88 patients from five Asian centers treated with sirolimus-coated stents, Nakamura and colleagues [30] reported a 6-month MACE rate of 4.5%, which were all target vessel revascularizations. The angiographic restenosis rate was only 3.4%. In the Sirolimus Eluting Stent in Chronic Total Occlusion study, 25 lesions were treated with sirolimus-coated stents. At 6-month follow-up only two patients (8%) had target vessel revascularization, and no other MACE was seen. Two studies of the use of paclitaxel-eluting stents have been reported. Werner and colleagues [31] presented the results of 48 patients who had CTO treated with the Taxus (Boston Scientific Corp., Natick, Massachusetts) stent and compared these results with historical controls using bare metal stents. There was an 84% reduction in the rate of restenosis (8.3% versus 51.1%; $P < .001$) and a 91% reduction in target vessel reocclusion (2.1% versus 23.4%; $P < .001$). The 1-year MACE rate was reduced by 74% (12.5% versus 47.9%; $P < .001$). The Wisdom registry reported the results in 65 patients who had CTO treated with TAXUS stents. At 12 months 6.7% of patients had any MACE, and these were all target vessel revascularizations, with one late stent thrombosis. Although the numbers are still small, and no controlled clinical trials have been conducted, there seems to be a striking reduction in cumulative late events to less than 10% when CTOs are treated with drug-eluting stents.

Summary

CTOs are prevalent in the coronary artery disease population but account for only 6% to

10% of coronary interventions. Clinical reasons to open CTOs include improved survival in those in whom the PCI is successful as well as improvement in angina, improved left ventricular function, and decreased need for CABG. Despite the high prevalence and clinical imperative to open CTOs, these patients continue to be the most problematic in interventional cardiology. Because of the nature of the pathobiology, these lesions are difficult to cross with a guidewire and sometimes with a balloon catheter. New guidewire technology has improved the success in crossing these lesions as well as the time required to cross. Some newer technology has improved the crossability of guidewire-refractory lesions. CTOs, however, still remain time consuming and difficult to open with low but sometimes significant acute complications. The restenosis rates and late occlusion rates are high. With the advent of stenting, there was a marked improvement in both late restenosis and late patency rates. Although the numbers are small, the use of drug-eluting stents has incrementally improved the long-term results with restenosis rates approaching 10% and late reocclusion rates in the low single-digit range.

References

[1] Stone G, Kandzari D, Mehran R, et al. Percutaneous recanalization of chronically occluded coronary arteries: a consensus document: part I. Circulation 2005;112:2364–72.

[2] Werner G, Emig U, Mutschke O, et al. Regression if collateral function after recanalization of chronic total coronary occlusions: a serial assessment by intracoronary pressure and Doppler recordings. Circulation 2003;108:2877–82.

[3] Tamai H, Berger P, Tsuchikane E, et al, for the Magic investigators. Frequency and time course of reocclusion and restenosis in coronary artery occlusions after balloon angioplasty versus Wiktor stent implantation. Am Heart J 2004;147:E9.

[4] Zidar F, Kaplan B, O'Neill W, et al. Prospective, randomized trial of prolonged intracoronary urokinase infusion for chronic total occlusions on native coronary arteries. J Am Coll Cardiol 1996;27: 1406–12.

[5] Olivari Z, Rubartelli P, Piscione F, et al, for the TOAST-GISE investigators. Immediate and one-year clinical outcome after percutaneous coronary interventions in chronic total occlusions: data from a multicenter, prospective, observational study (TOAST-GISE). J Am Coll Cardiol 2003;41:1672–8.

[6] King S, Lembo N, Weintraub W, et al. A randomized trial comparing coronary angioplasty with coronary bypass surgery. N Engl J Med 1994;331: 1044–50.

[7] Hoher M, Wohrle J, Grebe O, et al. A randomized trial of elective stenting after balloon recanalization of chronic total occlusions. J Am Coll Cardiol 1999; 34:722–9.

[8] Rubartelli P, Verna E, Niccoli L, et al, for the Gruppo Italiano de Studio sullo Stent nelle Occlusioni Coronariche investigators. Coronary stent implantation is superior to balloon angioplasty for chronic coronary occlusions: six-year clinical follow-up of the GISSOC trial. J Am Coll Cardiol 2003;41:1488–92.

[9] Buller C, Dzavik V, Carere R, et al. Primary stenting versus balloon angioplasty in occluded coronary arteries: the Total Occlusion Study of Canada (TOSCA). Circulation 1999;100:236–42.

[10] Kahn J. Angiographic suitability for catheter revascularization of total coronary occlusions in patients from a community hospital setting. Am Heart J 1993;126:561–4.

[11] Cohen H, Williams D, Holmes D, et al. Impact of age on procedural and 1-year outcome in percutaneous transluminal coronary angioplasty: the NHLBI Dynamic Registry. Am Heart J 2003;146:512–9.

[12] Hamm C, Reimers J, Ischinger T, et al, for the German Angioplasty Bypass Surgery Investigation. A randomized study of coronary angioplasty compared with bypass surgery in patients with symptomatic multivessel coronary disease. N Engl J Med 1994;331:1037–43.

[13] Bourassa M, Roubin G, Detre K, et al. Bypass Angioplasty Revascularization Investigation: patient screening, selection, and recruitment. Am J Cardiol 1995;75:3C–8C.

[14] Anderson H, Shaw R, Brindis R, et al. A contemporary overview of percutaneous coronary interventions: the American College of Cardiology-National Cardiovascular Data Registry (ACC-NCDR). J Am Coll Cardiol 2002;39:1096–103.

[15] Suero J, Marso S, Jones P, et al. Procedural outcomes and long-term survival among patients undergoing percutaneous coronary intervention of a chronic total occlusion in native coronary arteries: a 20-year experience. J Am Coll Cardiol 2001;38: 409–14.

[16] Ranmanathan K, Gao M, Nogareda G, et al. Successful percutaneous recanalization of a non-acute colluded coronary artery predicts clinical outcome and survival. Circulation 2001;104:II–415a.

[17] Hoye A, van Domburg R, Sonnenschein K, et al. Percutaneous coronary intervention for chronic total occlusions: the Thorax Center experience 1992–2002. Eur Heart J 2005;26:2630–6.

[18] Dzavik V, Caere R, Mancini G, et al, for the Total Occlusion Study of Canada Investigators. Predictors of improvement in left ventricular function after percutaneous revascularization of occluded coronary arteries. Am Heart J 2001;142:301–8.

[19] Simes P, Myreng Y, Malsted P, et al. Improvement of left ventricular ejection fraction and wall motion after successful recanalization of chronic coronary occlusions. Eur Heart J 1988;2:273–81.

[20] Chung C. Effect of recanalization of chronic total occlusions on global and regional left ventricular function in patients with and without previous myocardial infarction. Cath Cardiovasc Interv 2003; 60(3):368–74.

[21] Srivatsa S, Edwards W, Boos C, et al. Histologic correlates of angiographic chronic total coronary occlusions influence of occlusion duration an neovascular channel patterns an intimal plaque composition. J Am Coll Cardiol 1997;29:955–63.

[22] Katsuragawa M, Fujiware H, Miyamae M, et al. Histologic studies in percutaneous transluminal coronary angioplasty for chronic total occlusion: comparison of tapering and abrupt types of occlusion and short and long occluded segments. J Am Coll Cardiol 1993;21:604–11.

[23] Burke A, Kolodgie F, Farb A, et al. Morphological predictors of arterial remodeling in coronary atherosclerosis. Circulation 2002;105:297–303.

[24] Colombo A, Mikhail G, Michev I, et al. Treating chronic total occlusion using subintimal tracking and reentry: the STAR technique. Catheter Cardiovasc Interv 2005;64:407–11.

[25] Baim D, Braden G, Heuser R, et al. Utility of the Safe-Cross-guided radio frequency total occlusion crossing system in chronic coronary total occlusions. Am J Cardiol 2004;94:853–8.

[26] Whitlow P, Selmon M, O'Neill W, et al. Treatment of uncrossable chronic total coronary occlusions with the Frontrunner: multicenter experience. J Am Coll Cardiol 2002;90:168H.

[27] Michalis L, Rees M, Davis J, et al. Use of vibrational angioplasty for the treatment of chronic total coronary occlusions. Catheter Cardiovasc Interv 1999; 46:98–104.

[28] Serruys P, Hamburger J, Koolen J, et al. Total occlusion trial with angioplasty by using laser guidewire. Eur Heart J 2000;21:1797–805.

[29] Hoye A, Tanabe K, Lemos P, et al. Significant reduction in restenosis after the use of sirolimus-eluting stents in the treatment of chronic total occlusions. J Am Coll Cardiol 2004;43:1954–8.

[30] Nakamura S, Selvan TS, Bae JH, et al. Impact of sirolimus-eluting stents on the outcome of patients with chronic total occlusions: multicenter registry in Asia. J Am Coll Cardiol 2004;43:35A.

[31] Werner GS, Krack A, Schwarz G, et al. Prevention of lesion recurrence in chronic total coronary occlusions by paclitaxel-eluting stents. J Am Coll Cardiol 2004;44:2301–6.

ELSEVIER
SAUNDERS

Cardiol Clin 24 (2006) 255–263

CARDIOLOGY
CLINICS

Percutaneous Coronary Interventions: Guidelines, Short- and Long-Term Results, and Comparison with Coronary Artery Bypass Grafting

Joaquin E. Cigarroa, MD, L. David Hillis, MD*

Department of Internal Medicine, Cardiovascular Division, University of Texas Southwestern Medical Center, 5323 Harry Hines Boulevard, Dallas, TX 75390-9030, USA

In the United States and throughout the western world, the prevalence of ischemic heart disease is high due to a relatively high incidence among the population of advanced age, obesity, and certain risk factors for atherosclerosis (most notably hypertension and diabetes mellitus). The widespread use of noninvasive testing for identifying those who are likely to have coronary artery disease (ie, exercise testing with or without echocardiographic or radionuclide imaging and the more recently developed MRI and CT angiography) has resulted in a substantial increase in the number of patients undergoing diagnostic coronary angiography, which in turn has resulted in an increased number of individuals who are referred for percutaneous or surgical coronary revascularization. In the United States in 2002, according to the American Heart Association, approximately 1.2 million people had a percutaneous coronary intervention (PCI) and 0.5 million underwent coronary artery bypass grafting (CABG). In individuals who have coronary artery disease, coronary revascularization may be performed (1) to reduce morbidity by eliminating or reducing anginal frequency and severity or, on occasion, by alleviating symptoms of heart failure (dyspnea or fatigue); or (2) to reduce mortality in selected patient subsets. The decision to proceed with percutaneous or surgical revascularization should be based on a thorough and complete understanding of the short- and long-term risks and benefits of each procedure in conjunction with the individual patient's coronary arterial anatomy and clinical risk profile.

Coronary artery bypass grafting

CABG was first reported in 1969 by Favaloro [1]. Subsequent randomized comparisons in the 1970s of CABG and medical therapy in subjects who had stable or unstable angina [2–6] established the superiority of surgical revascularization in relieving angina, improving exercise tolerance, and reducing the need for antianginal medications. In addition, apart from symptom relief, CABG was superior to medical therapy in improving survival in subjects who had (1) three-vessel coronary artery disease and a left ventricular ejection fraction less than 0.50, (2) two- or three-vessel coronary artery disease in which the proximal left anterior descending coronary artery was significantly narrowed [4], and (3) left main coronary artery disease.

Percutaneous coronary intervention

The first PCI was reported by Gruntzig and colleagues in 1979 [7]. Over the next several years, substantial improvements in equipment, including the design and manufacture of guiding catheters, guidewires, and balloon catheters, led to the use of this therapeutic modality in a growing number of patients so that by the mid- to late-1980s, its use was widespread. Small randomized trials demonstrated that PCI was superior to medical

* Corresponding author.
E-mail address: dhilli@parknet.pmh.org
(L.D. Hillis).

therapy in the alleviation of angina [8]. At the same time, these studies failed to demonstrate that PCI reduced the occurrence of subsequent ischemic events or death and established the relatively high incidence (35%–40%) of a required repeat revascularization procedure during the subsequent year in patients whose initial PCI had been successful, a process known as restenosis. The procedural success and safety of PCI in patients who had single-vessel coronary artery disease led to its application in patients who had multivessel disease. Subsequently, the growing use of PCI in this patient population led to the performance of randomized comparisons of PCI and CABG [9–17].

Coronary artery bypass grafting versus percutaneous coronary intervention in patients who have stable or unstable angina

Coronary artery bypass grafting versus percutaneous transluminal coronary angioplasty

From the mid-1980s to the mid-1990s, nine randomized comparisons of CABG and percutaneous transluminal coronary angioplasty (PTCA; balloon angioplasty) in patients who had single- or multivessel coronary artery disease were reported—all of which produced remarkably similar and consistent results [9–17]. First, the two methods of revascularization were associated with a similarly low periprocedural mortality (1.0%–1.5%). Second, the periprocedural morbidity that occurred with CABG was higher (the incidence of periprocedural Q wave myocardial infarction ranged from 4.6% to 10.3% with CABG and only 2.1% to 6.3% with PTCA) and the length of hospital stay was longer with CABG than with PTCA. Third, those who underwent CABG experienced more effective relief of angina. As a result, they had less need for antianginal medications and were less likely to require a repeat revascularization procedure. Lastly, long-term survival was similar for the two treatment strategies.

A subsequent analysis of the results of the largest of these trials, the Bypass Angioplasty Revascularization Investigation (BARI) [14], strongly suggested that long-term survival was better with CABG than with PTCA in patients who had treated diabetes mellitus, whereas survival with the two treatment strategies was similar in those who did not have treated diabetes mellitus. In BARI [14], 1829 patients who had (1)

angina or other evidence of myocardial ischemia, (2) multivessel coronary artery disease, and (3) coronary arterial anatomic features that made them eligible for either procedure were randomly assigned to receive CABG (n = 914) or PTCA (n = 915) (Table 1).

Of the 914 patients who were assigned to receive CABG, 98% received it. All intended vessels were grafted in 91% of patients, and in 82%, the left internal mammary artery was used as one of the conduits. The median hospital stay following CABG was 7 days. Of the 915 patients assigned to receive PTCA, 99% received it. Balloon angioplasty of multiple coronary arterial stenoses was attempted in 78% of patients and resulted in an average of 1.9 of 3.5 (54%) clinically important stenoses dilated successfully. The median hospital stay after PTCA was 3 days.

With both treatment modalities, the in-hospital mortality was less than 1.5% (Table 2). PTCA resulted in a lower incidence of periprocedural Q wave myocardial infarction (2.1% for PTCA, 4.5% for CABG, $P < 0.01$) but was accompanied by the need for more subsequent urgent revascularization procedures (8.3% for PTCA, 0.1% for CABG, $P < 0.001$) and nonurgent revascularization procedures (5.1% for PTCA, 0% for

Table 1
Characteristics of the patients assigned to undergo percutaneous transluminal coronary angioplasty or coronary artery bypass grafting in the Bypass Angioplasty Revascularization Investigation

Characteristic	CABG (n = 914)	PTCA (n = 915)
Mean age (y)	61.1	61.8
Female sex (%)	26	27
Previous myocardial infarction (%)	55	54
Congestive heart failure (%)	9	9
Treated diabetes mellitus (%)	25	24
Unstable angina (%)	65	63
Three-vessel CAD (%)	41	41
Proximal LAD involvement (%)	37	36
LV ejection fraction <0.50 (%)	21	23

Abbreviations: CAD, coronary artery disease; LAD, left anterior descending; LV, left ventricular.

Data from Comparison of coronary bypass surgery with angioplasty in patients with multivessel disease. The Bypass Angioplasty Revascularization Investigation (BARI) investigators. N Engl J Med 1996;335:219.

Table 2

In-hospital complications of coronary artery bypass grafting and percutaneous transluminal coronary angioplasty in the Bypass Angioplasty Revascularization Investigation

Complication	CABG (n = 914)	PTCA (n = 915)
Death	12 (1.3%)	10 (1.1%)
Q wave MI	41 (4.5%)	19 (2.1%)*
Death/Q wave MI	52 (5.7%)	27 (3.0%)*
Urgent CABG	1 (0.1%)	57 (6.2%)**
Urgent PTCA	0	19 (2.1%)**
Stroke	7 (0.8%)	2 (0.2%)
Nonurgent CABG/PTCA	0	47 (5.1%)**

Abbreviation: MI, myocardial infarction.

* $P < 0.01$; ** $P < 0.001$ in comparison to CABG.

Data from Comparison of coronary bypass surgery with angioplasty in patients with multivessel disease. The Bypass Angioplasty Revascularization Investigation (BARI) investigators. N Engl J Med 1996;335:220.

Table 3

Results of the Bypass Angioplasty Revascularization Investigation

Result	CABG (n = 914)	PTCA (n = 915)
In-hospital mortality	1.3%	1.1%
Periprocedural Q wave MI	4.5%	2.1%*
Periprocedural stroke	0.8%	0.2%
5-y survival (all patients)	89.3%	86.3%
5-y survival free of MI	80.4%	78.7%
Repeat revascularization within 5 y	8.0%	54.0%**
5-y survival (treated diabetics)	80.6%	65.5%***

Abbreviation: MI, myocardial infarction.

* $P < 0.01$; ** $P < 0.001$; *** $P < 0.003$ in comparison to CABG.

Data from Comparison of coronary bypass surgery with angioplasty in patients with multivessel disease. The Bypass Angioplasty Revascularization Investigation (BARI) investigators. N Engl J Med 1996;335:220.

CABG, $P < 0.001$). Procedural morbidity including respiratory failure, reoperation for bleeding, and wound infection was higher for CABG (9.4% for CABG, 1.8% for PTCA, $P < 0.001$). In summary, CABG and PTCA were accompanied by a low periprocedural mortality. In comparison to PTCA, CABG achieved more complete revascularization, thereby resulting in less need for antianginal medications and repeat revascularization procedures, but was associated with a higher incidence of periprocedural Q wave myocardial infarction and a longer length of hospital stay (see Table 2).

The 1829 subjects enrolled in BARI were followed for an average of 5.4 years (Table 3). In comparison to those who had CABG, those who had PTCA were more likely to require a repeat revascularization procedure during this period of follow-up (54% for PTCA, 8% for CABG, $P < 0.001$). The incidence of myocardial infarction and death was similar for the two treatment strategies (myocardial infarction: 21% for CABG, 20% for PTCA, not significant [NS]; death: 14% for CABG, 11% for PTCA, NS). In patients who were undergoing treatment for diabetes mellitus, a post hoc analysis revealed a substantial survival advantage with CABG (total mortality 19.4% for CABG, 34.5% for PTCA, $P < 0.003$).

Subsequent analyses of "registry data" from nonrandomized groups of patients who had multivessel coronary artery disease and diabetes

mellitus have provided mixed results in comparison to the results of the BARI randomized trial. Similar to BARI, some of these analyses demonstrated a survival advantage of CABG over PTCA in this patient population [18], whereas others showed that this population's long-term mortality was similar with CABG or with PTCA [19]. Even the nonrandomized registry data from the BARI investigators showed no difference in long-term mortality between the two treatment groups [20]. These disparate results are likely due to differences in coronary anatomy between the patients enrolled in the registry and those in the randomized trial.

As noted, previously published studies have demonstrated that CABG is superior to medical therapy in improving survival in patients who had three-vessel coronary artery disease and a left ventricular ejection fraction less than 0.50 [2,3] and who had two- or three-vessel coronary artery disease with normal left ventricular systolic function if the proximal left anterior descending coronary artery is significantly narrowed [4]. Are the long-term results of PTCA similar to those of CABG in these specific patient populations? The answer appears to be yes. Berger and colleagues [21] examined the results of BARI in patients who had these specific anatomic features and who did not have diabetes mellitus and provided actuarial survival data over a period of observation of 7 years. For all patients who had three-vessel coronary artery disease, survival was similar at 7 years for CABG (87%) and PTCA (85%) (Fig. 1). For those who had three-vessel coronary artery disease and a left ventricular ejection fraction less than 0.50, survival at 7 years for CABG or PTCA was similar (73% for CABG, 82% for PTCA, NS) (Fig. 2). For patients who had two-vessel coronary artery disease and significant narrowing of the proximal left anterior descending coronary artery, survival at 7 years was similar for the two treatment groups (86% for CABG, 93% for PTCA, NS) (Fig. 3). Finally, for those who had two-vessel coronary artery disease involving the proximal left anterior descending coronary artery and a left ventricular ejection fraction less than 0.50, survival at 7 years was statistically similar for those undergoing CABG and PTCA (67% and 90%, respectively, NS) (Fig. 4).

In summary, the nine randomized comparisons of CABG and PTCA [9–17] showed that (1) the two procedures are associated with a similar periprocedural and long-term mortality, but the data from the randomized portion of BARI suggest strongly that long-term survival is better with CABG in patients who have treated diabetes mellitus; and (2) although CABG is accompanied by greater periprocedural morbidity, it affords greater angina relief and less of a need for subsequent urgent and elective repeat revascularization procedures.

Coronary artery bypass grafting versus stenting

By the mid-1990s, intracoronary stenting had largely supplanted PTCA in most patients undergoing percutaneous coronary revascularization. In comparison to PTCA, stenting offers several advantages including (1) a reduced incidence of symptomatic restenosis (35%–40% with PTCA, 20%–25% with stenting); (2) a reduced need for urgent CABG; and (3) a decreased procedural time. The acceptance of intracoronary stenting as the preferred method of PCI led to several randomized comparisons of stenting and CABG in patients who had single- and multivessel coronary artery disease [22–25].

From April 1997 to June 1998, Serruys and colleagues [23] randomly assigned 1205 patients who had stable or unstable angina and multivessel coronary artery disease to CABG (n = 605) or stenting (n = 600). Two thirds of the patients had two-vessel coronary artery disease and the remainder had three-vessel disease. Only 4% of subjects had an occluded (as opposed to narrowed) major epicardial coronary artery. Of the patients who were randomly assigned to stenting, an average of 2.8 coronary arterial stenoses were noted on angiography, and an average of 2.6 of these were stented (in 89%) or dilated with a balloon (in 11%). Of the individuals randomly assigned to undergo CABG, an average of 2.8 coronary

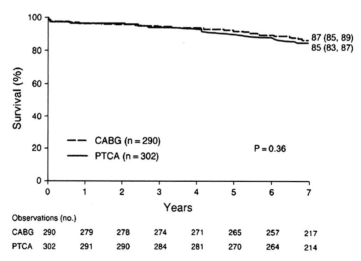

Fig. 1. Actuarial survival, in years, expressed as a percentage, in nondiabetic patients who had three-vessel coronary artery disease. At 7 years, the survival in those undergoing CABG and PTCA was similar. (*From* Berger PB, Velianou JL, Aslanidou Vlachos H, et al. Survival following coronary angioplasty versus coronary artery bypass surgery in anatomic subsets in which coronary artery bypass surgery improves survival compared with medical therapy. Results from the Bypass Angioplasty Revascularization Investigation (BARI). J Am Coll Cardiol 2001;38:1445; with permission.)

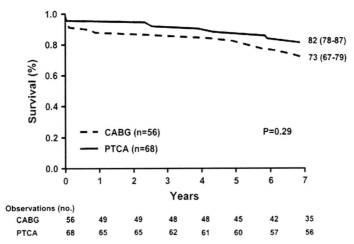

Fig. 2. Actuarial survival, in years, expressed as a percentage, in nondiabetic patients who had three-vessel coronary artery disease and depressed left ventricular systolic function. At 7 years, the survival in those having CABG and PTCA was similar. (*From* Berger PB, Velianou JL, Aslanidou Vlachos H, et al. Survival following coronary angioplasty versus coronary artery bypass surgery in anatomic subsets in which coronary artery bypass surgery improves survival compared with medical therapy. Results from the Bypass Angioplasty Revascularization Investigation (BARI). J Am Coll Cardiol 2001;38:1445; with permission.)

arterial stenoses were noted, and these patients received an average of 2.5 conduits; 93% of this group received at least one arterial conduit.

In comparison to those undergoing stenting, the patients treated with CABG had a higher incidence of periprocedural myocardial infarction, defined as a rise in serum MB fraction of creatine kinase (CK-MB) greater than five times the upper limit of normal (12.6% for CABG, 6.2% for stenting, $P < 0.001$). The incidence of subsequent unplanned revascularization procedures was statistically similar (0.3% for CABG, 2.3% for

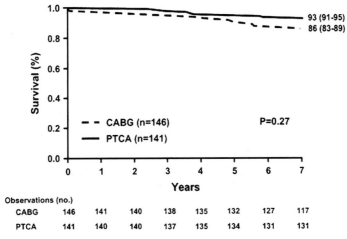

Fig. 3. Actuarial survival, in years, expressed as a percentage, in nondiabetic patients who had two-vessel coronary artery disease and significant narrowing of the proximal left anterior descending coronary artery. At 7 years, the survival in those undergoing CABG and PTCA was similar. (*From* Berger PB, Velianou JL, Aslanidou Vlachos H, et al. Survival following coronary angioplasty versus coronary artery bypass surgery in anatomic subsets in which coronary artery bypass surgery improves survival compared with medical therapy. Results from the Bypass Angioplasty Revascularization Investigation (BARI). J Am Coll Cardiol 2001;38:1447; with permission.)

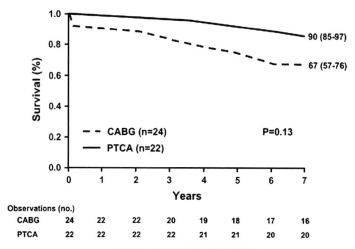

Fig. 4. Actuarial survival, in years, expressed as a percentage, in nondiabetic patients who had two-vessel coronary artery disease, significant narrowing of the proximal left anterior descending coronary artery, and depressed left ventricular systolic function. At 7 years, the survival in those having CABG and PTCA was similar. (*From* Berger PB, Velianou JL, Aslanidou Vlachos H, et al. Survival following coronary angioplasty versus coronary artery bypass surgery in anatomic subsets in which coronary artery bypass surgery improves survival compared with medical therapy. Results from the Bypass Angioplasty Revascularization Investigation (BARI). J Am Coll Cardiol 2001;38:1447; with permission.)

stenting, NS). During the first month after stenting, subacute stent thrombosis occurred in 2.8%.

As shown in Table 4, the incidence of death, stroke, and myocardial infarction was similar in the two treatment groups 1 year after randomization. During this first year of observation, however, those who had stenting were more likely to require a second revascularization procedure (21.0% for stenting, 3.8% for CABG, $P<0.01$). The patients who received CABG were more likely to be free of angina (89.5% for CABG, 78.9% for stenting, $P<0.001$).

As displayed in Table 5, the data acquired after 5 years of follow-up demonstrate that the subjects who had stenting were more likely than those who

had CABG to experience an adverse outcome, defined as the occurrence of death, myocardial infarction, stroke, or a repeat revascularization procedure. Specifically, in the 5 years following randomization, 78.2% of those who underwent CABG had none of these adverse outcomes, whereas only 58.3% of those who had stenting were free of them ($P<0.001$). This difference between the two treatment groups was largely driven by the substantial difference in the need for a repeat revascularization procedure in those undergoing stenting (41.7% for stenting, 21.8% for

Table 4
Arterial Revascularization Therapies I trial 1-y outcomes: coronary artery bypass grafting versus stenting

Outcome	CABG (n = 605)	Stenting (n = 600)
Death	2.8%	2.5%
Cerebrovascular accident	2.1%	1.7%
Myocardial infarction	4.8%	6.2%
Repeat Revascularization	3.8%	21.0%[*]

* $P<0.01$ in comparison to CABG.

Data from Serruys PW, Unger F, Sousa JE, et al. Comparison of coronary-artery bypass surgery and stenting for the treatment of multivessel disease. N Engl J Med 2001;344:1119.

Table 5
Arterial Revascularization Therapies I trial 5-y outcomes: coronary artery bypass grafting versus stenting

Outcome	CABG (n = 605)	Stenting (n = 600)
Freedom from death/MI/ CVA/revascularization	78.2%	58.3%[*]
Death	7.6%	8.0%
Repeat revascularization	21.8%	41.7%[*]
Angina	15.5%	21.2%

Abbreviations: CVA, cerebrovascular accident; MI, myocardial infarction.

* $P<0.001$ in comparison to CABG.

Data from Serruys PW, Unger F, Sousa JE, et al. Comparison of coronary-artery bypass surgery and stenting for the treatment of multivessel disease. N Engl J Med 2001;344:1119.

CABG, $P < 0.001$). During the 5 years of observation, mortality was similar in the two groups (7.6% for CABG, 8.0% for stenting, NS), as was the likelihood of continued angina (21.2% for stenting, 15.5% for CABG, NS) and the need for antianginal medications.

Serruys and colleagues [23] studied the monetary costs of the two treatment strategies. The cost of the initial procedure averaged $4212 less for stenting than for CABG ($6441 for stenting, $10,653 for CABG). Although this advantage in favor of stenting persisted at 1 year, eventually it was reduced in magnitude (to $2973 per patient) due to a greater need for repeat revascularization procedures in the stented group. Similar short- and long-term cost advantages of stenting over CABG have been shown to be present in the Stent or Surgery Trial [26].

In summary, the randomized comparisons of CABG and coronary stenting provided the following results. First, the two procedures were associated with a similar periprocedural and long-term mortality. Second, although CABG was accompanied by greater periprocedural morbidity, it afforded better angina relief and less need for subsequent urgent or elective repeat revascularization procedures. Third, those who had stenting had a shorter length of hospital stay and a smaller hospital bill. In comparison to PTCA, coronary stenting improves the completeness of revascularization, reduces the need for urgent CABG, and decreases the need for subsequent revascularization by decreasing the incidence of restenosis. In addition, stenting provides the operator with the ability to address complex coronary arterial stenoses (ie, those that are particularly long or angulated and those located at a coronary arterial bifurcation) with less uncertainty in the outcome.

In all the previously cited comparisons of CABG and PCI, the consistent (and only) disadvantage of the latter has been the substantial percentage of patients who have recurrent symptoms in the weeks to months after the initially successful procedure, thereby requiring repeat coronary angiography and, in most individuals, an additional revascularization procedure (CABG or repeat PCI). The recurrence of symptoms is usually caused by restenosis at the site of previous balloon dilatation or stent deployment. As stated previously, symptomatic restenosis occurs in about 35% of patients in the 12 months after successful PTCA and in 20% to 25% of those who have had successful stenting. If one could effectively prevent restenosis, this one major disadvantage of PCI would be alleviated, thereby making PCI more attractive than CABG (provided that contraindications to PCI do not exist). Recently published data [26] demonstrate that the use of sirolimus-eluting stents dramatically reduces the incidence of restenosis. Specifically, of 238 patients randomly assigned to receive a standard (n = 118) or a sirolimus-eluting (n = 120) stent, 27% of the former and 0% of the latter group developed restenosis within 6 months of the procedure ($P < 0.001$). These striking results await confirmation in studies of patients who have multivessel coronary artery disease. The results of the Arterial Revascularization Therapies II trial, a nonrandomized open-label registry that compared the results of drug-eluting stent deployment in 607 subjects with the results obtained in a group of individuals who underwent CABG and whose outcomes were described previously in the literature (so-called "historical controls"), suggest that the two procedures are accompanied by a similar incidence of myocardial infarction, required repeat revascularization procedures, and death during 1 year of observation (Table 6) [27].

Limitations of randomized trials comparing coronary artery bypass grafting and percutaneous coronary intervention

The multiple randomized trials comparing CABG and PCI described previously have

Table 6
Arterial Revascularization Therapies II trial 1-y clinical outcomes

Outcome	Drug-eluting stents (n = 607)	CABG (n = 605)
Death	1.0%	2.7%
MI	1.2%	3.5%
Cerebrovascular accident	0.8%	1.8%
CABG	2.0%	0.7%
PCI	5.4%	3.0%
Death/MI/CVA/ revascularization	10.4%	11.6%

Abbreviations: CVA, cerebrovascular accident; MI, myocardial infarction.
Data from Serruys PW. Preliminary results of the second Arterial Revascularization Therapy Study trial (ARTS II). Presented at the American College of Cardiology Annual Scientific Sessions, March 6, 2005, Orlando, Florida.

provided valuable insights into the relative benefits and limitations of each procedure. By eliminating (or at least minimizing) physician and
patient "selection bias," these trials help to ensure
that patient comorbidities and concurrent management strategies are distributed similarly between the two revascularization techniques.
Nonetheless, they have limitations. First, only
a small fraction (5%–12%) of patients who were
evaluated for possible enrollment in these randomized trails were found to be eligible; therefore,
the results may not be easily generalized and
applicable to the much larger group of patients
requiring revascularization (most of whom would
have been ineligible for enrollment). Second, most
of these randomized trials were not of sufficient
statistical power to allow definitive conclusions
regarding survival. Data from large registries,
although not randomized, avoid the aforemen-
tioned potential limitations of randomized trials.
In this regard, the results of the New York
Registry, recently reported by Hannan and colleagues [28], are of considerable interest. In this
analysis of data from almost 60,000 patients
who had multivessel coronary artery disease undergoing CABG (n = 37,212) or PCI (n =
22,102) between January 1997 and December
2000, those with two- or three-vessel disease had
a better long-term survival with CABG than
with PCI. The survival advantage of CABG over
PCI was demonstrable in all patient subgroups
who had multivessel coronary artery disease, irrespective of (1) the location of the stenosis in the
left anterior descending coronary artery (proximal
or nonproximal); (2) the presence or absence of diabetes mellitus; and (3) left ventricular systolic
function.

Implications for patient management

The management of the patient who has
(1) single-vessel coronary artery disease (regardless
of left ventricular systolic function); (2) two-vessel
disease not involving the proximal left anterior
descending coronary artery (regardless of left
ventricular systolic function); and (3) three-vessel
disease and normal left ventricular systolic function can be individualized and "symptom-driven."
For some of these patients, medical therapy will
suffice, in that it will substantially or completely
alleviate symptoms. When nonmedical treatment
is chosen, the decision of whether to use percutaneous or surgical revascularization should be
reached "with the understanding that CABG is

associated with greater initial morbidity but results
in more effective relief of angina and freedom from
repeat procedures in the ensuing years. On the
other hand, PCI is associated with a lower rate of
initial morbidity but a greater likelihood of recurrent angina, need for antianginal medications,
and subsequent revascularization procedures"
[29]. The use of drug-eluting stents is likely to reduce the need for subsequent revascularization
procedures.

The patient who has three-vessel coronary
artery disease and depressed left ventricular systolic function (ejection fraction <0.50) or two- or
three-vessel disease with narrowing of the proximal left anterior descending coronary artery (regardless of left ventricular systolic function)
should be encouraged to undergo percutaneous
or surgical revascularization (irrespective of symptoms) to achieve an improved survival. If the
patient is diabetic, then CABG is probably preferred (based on the results of the randomized
portion of BARI). If the patient is not diabetic
and his or her coronary anatomy is amenable to
either therapeutic strategy, then the decision of
whether to use percutaneous or surgical therapy
can be based on the patient's preferences, with
appropriate input from his or her physician.

References

[1] Favaloro RG. Saphenous vein graft in the surgical
    treatment of coronary artery disease. Operative
    technique. J Thorac Cardiovasc Surg 1969;58:
    178–85.
[2] The Veterans administration Coronary artery
    Bypass Surgery Cooperative Study Group. Eleven-
    year survival in the Veterans Administration ran-
    domized trial of coronary bypass surgery for stable
    angina. The Veterans Administration Coronary
    Artery Bypass Surgery Cooperative Study Group.
    N Engl J Med 1984;311:1333–9.
[3] Alderman EL, Bourassa MG, Cohen LS, et al. Ten-
    year follow-up of survival and myocardial infarction
    in the randomized Coronary Artery Surgery Study.
    Circulation 1990;82:1629–46.
[4] Varnauskas E. Twelve-year follow-up of survival in
    the randomized European Coronary Surgery Study.
    N Engl J Med 1988;319:332–7.
[5] Booth DC, Deupree RH, Hultgren HN, et al.
    Quality of life after bypass surgery for unstable
    angina. 5-year follow-up results of a Veterans Affairs
    Cooperative Study. Circulation 1991;83:87–95.
[6] Russell RO Jr, Moraski RE, Kouchoukos N, et al.
    Unstable angina pectoris: National Cooperative
    Study Group to Compare Surgical and Medical
    Therapy. Am J Cardiol 1978;42:839–48.

[7] Gruntzig AR, Senning A, Siegenthaler WE. Nonoperative dilatation of coronary-artery stenosis: percutaneous transluminal coronary angioplasty. N Engl J Med 1979;301:61–8.

[8] Parisi AF, Folland ED, Hartigan P. A comparison of angioplasty with medical therapy in the treatment of single-vessel coronary artery disease. Veterans Affairs ACME Investigators. N Engl J Med 1992;326:10–6.

[9] RITA Trial Participants. Coronary angioplasty versus coronary artery bypass surgery: the Randomized Intervention Treatment of Angina (RITA) trial. Lancet 1993;341:573–80.

[10] Rodriguez A, Boullon F, Perez-Balino N, et al. Argentine randomized trial of percutaneous transluminal coronary angioplasty versus coronary artery bypass surgery in multivessel disease (ERACI): in-hospital results and 1-year follow-up. ERACI Group. J Am Coll Cardiol 1993;22:1060–7.

[11] Hamm CW, Reimers J, Ischinger T, et al. A randomized study of coronary angioplasty compared with bypass surgery in patients with symptomatic multivessel coronary disease. German Angioplasty Bypass Surgery Investigation (GABI). N Engl J Med 1994;331:1037–43.

[12] King III SB, Lembo NJ, Weintraub WS, et al. A randomized trial comparing coronary angioplasty with coronary bypass surgery. Emory Angioplasty versus Surgery Trial (EAST). N Engl J Med 1994; 331:1044–50.

[13] CABRI Trial Participants. First-year results of CABRI (Coronary Angioplasty versus Bypass Revascularisation Investigation). CABRI Trial Participants. Lancet 1995;346:1179–84.

[14] The Bypass angioplasty Revascularization Investigation (BARI) Investigators. Comparison of coronary bypass surgery with angioplasty in patients with multivessel disease. The Bypass Angioplasty Revascularization Investigation (BARI) investigators. N Engl J Med 1996;335:217–25.

[15] Goy JJ, Eeckhout E, Burnand B, et al. Coronary angioplasty versus left internal mammary artery grafting for isolated proximal left anterior descending artery stenosis. Lancet 1994;343:1449–53.

[16] Carrie D, Elbaz M, Puel J, et al. Five-year outcome after coronary angioplasty versus bypass surgery in multivessel coronary artery disease: results from the French Monocentric Study. Circulation 1997;96:II-1–6.

[17] Hueb WA, Bellotti G, de Oliveira SA, et al. The Medicine, Angioplasty or Surgery Study (MASS): a prospective, randomized trial of medical therapy, balloon angioplasty or bypass surgery for single proximal left anterior descending artery stenoses. J Am Coll Cardiol 1995;26:1600–5.

[18] Niles NW, McGrath PD, Malenka D, et al. Survival of patients with diabetes and multivessel coronary artery disease after surgical or percutaneous coronary revascularization: results of a large regional prospective study. Northern New England Cardiovascular Disease Study Group. J Am Coll Cardiol 2001;37:1008–15.

[19] Barsness GW, Peterson ED, Ohman EM, et al. Relationship between diabetes mellitus and long-term survival after coronary bypass and angioplasty. Circulation 1997;96:2551–6.

[20] Detre KM, Guo P, Holubkov R, et al. Coronary revascularization in diabetic patients: a comparison of the randomized and observational components of the Bypass Angioplasty Revascularization Investigation (BARI). Circulation 1999;99:633–40.

[21] Berger PB, Velianou JL, Aslanidou Vlachos H, et al. Survival following coronary angioplasty versus coronary artery bypass surgery in anatomic subsets in which coronary artery bypass surgery improves survival compared with medical therapy. Results from the Bypass Angioplasty Revascularization Investigation (BARI). J Am Coll Cardiol 2001;38:1440–9.

[22] Hueb W, Soares PR, Gersh BJ, et al. The medicine, angioplasty, or surgery study (MASS-II): a randomized, controlled clinical trial of three therapeutic strategies for multivessel coronary artery disease: one-year results. J Am Coll Cardiol 2004;43:1743–51.

[23] Serruys PW, Unger F, Sousa JE, et al. Comparison of coronary-artery bypass surgery and stenting for the treatment of multivessel disease. N Engl J Med 2001;344:1117–24.

[24] The SOS Investigators. Coronary artery bypass surgery versus percutaneous coronary intervention with stent implantation in patients with multivessel coronary artery disease (the Stent or Surgery trial): a randomised controlled trial. Lancet 2002;360:965–70.

[25] Rodriguez A, Bernardi V, Navia J, et al. Argentine randomized study: coronary angioplasty with stenting versus coronary bypass surgery in patients with multiple-vessel disease (ERACI II): 30-day and one-year follow-up results. ERACI II Investigators. J Am Coll Cardiol 2001;37:51–8.

[26] Weintraub WS, Mahoney EM, Zhang Z, et al. One year comparison of costs of coronary surgery versus percutaneous coronary intervention in the stent or surgery trial. Heart 2004;90:782–8.

[27] Serruys PW, for the ARTS-II Investigators. ARTS-II: Arterial Revascularization Therapies Study Part II of the sirolimus-eluting stent in the treatment of patients with multivessel de novo coronary artery lesions. Late Breaking Clinical Trial. Presented at the American College of Cardiology 54th Annual Meeting: Orlando, FL; March 2005.

[28] Hannan EL, Racz MJ, Walford G, et al. Long-term outcomes of coronary-artery bypass grafting versus stent implantation. N Engl J Med 2005;352:2174–83.

[29] Hillis LD, Rutherford JD. Coronary angioplasty compared with bypass grafting. N Engl J Med 1994;331:1086–7.

Percutaneous Left Ventricular Support Devices

Michael S. Lee, MD, Raj R. Makkar, MD*

*Cardiovascular Intervention Center, Cedars-Sinai Medical Center, University of California,
Los Angeles School of Medicine, 8631 West Third Street, Room 415E, Los Angeles, CA 90048, USA*

Patients in cardiogenic shock or patients who have left ventricular dysfunction or complex coronary lesions such as multivessel coronary disease, bypass graft disease, or left main disease who undergo percutaneous coronary intervention (PCI) are at increased risk of adverse outcomes from detrimental hemodynamic effects due to ischemia from balloon inflations, dissection, abrupt vessel closure, malignant arrhythmias, or "no reflow" [1–3]. Left ventricular assist devices (LVADs) have been used as therapeutic instruments for cardiac insufficiency including left ventricular failure, cardiogenic shock, and low cardiac output syndrome and as a bridge to transplantation. Percutaneous LVADs have long been of major interest to operators to provide partial or total hemodynamic support to patients in cardiogenic shock and during high-risk PCI without the need for surgical implantation.

Expedient initiation of percutaneous circulatory support may provide hemodynamic stability during high-risk PCI. Percutaneous LVADs through the femoral approach have been developed to provide circulatory support during high-risk PCI by withdrawing oxygenated blood from the left heart into systemic circulation [4–6]. Current percutaneous LVADs include the Tandem-Heart (CardiacAssist, Pittsburgh, Pennsylvania) and the Impella Recover LP 2.5 System (Impella CardioSystems, Aachen, Germany), which can be inserted under fluoroscopy in the cardiac catheterization laboratory without the need for extracorporeal oxygenation and surgical implantation

and provide temporary hemodynamic stabilization during high-risk PCI. In this article, the authors review the current percutaneous LVADs available for circulatory support.

Cardiogenic shock, which occurs in 7% to 10% of cases after acute myocardial infarction, is the most common cause of in-hospital death in patients who have acute myocardial infarction [7]. The intra-aortic balloon pump (IABP) can augment coronary perfusion in cardiogenic shock and high-risk PCI patients but provides minimal circulatory support in the setting of complete hemodynamic collapse and minimal benefit in mortality [8,9]. The LVAD markedly reduced the extent of myocardial necrosis in animal models of acute myocardial infarction [10–12]. The routine use of the LVAD in acute myocardial infarction and cardiogenic shock is not practical because the surgical implantation of the LVAD requires a midline sternotomy [13]. Furthermore, patients who had acute myocardial infarction who required temporary circulatory support with an LVAD had a very high mortality rate [14].

With the improvement of device technology and adjunctive pharmacotherapy, interventional cardiologists are tackling more complex and high-risk PCI cases. LVADs provide hemodynamic support during high-risk PCI, especially during balloon inflation, by unloading the left ventricle and augmenting systemic circulation. One of the earlier devices used to provide circulatory support during elective PCI was the femorofemoral cardiopulmonary support system, which required a perfusionist to direct the system [15]. With "supported angioplasty," the femorofemoral cardiopulmonary support system was associated with complications at the cannula site, including

* Corresponding author.
E-mail address: raj.makkar@cshs.org
(R.R. Makkar).

0733-8651/06/$ - see front matter © 2006 Elsevier Inc. All rights reserved.
doi:10.1016/j.ccl.2006.01.004

vascular complications, femoral neuropathy, skin infection, and skin necrosis. These complications occurred in equal frequency in percutaneous and cut-down cannulation. Thirty percent of patients required blood transfusions, perhaps because the activated clotting time required to maintain the system was greater than 400 seconds [16]. Another LVAD, the Hemopump Cardiac Assist System (Medtronic, Minneapolis, Minnesota), is no longer used today because of increased morbidity and mortality due to large arterial cannulae, hemolysis, thromboembolism, and the need for anesthetists and perfusionists [17,18]. Since then, the TandemHeart percutaneous LVAD and the Impella Recover LP 2.5 System have been introduced to provide circulatory support during high-risk PCI (Table 1).

Intra-aortic balloon pump

The IABP was first used clinically for supporting patients who had cardiogenic shock after acute myocardial infarction [19]. Since then, its use has continued to increase in a variety of settings, including providing mechanical assistance in patients who have hemodynamic instability during PCI. The IABP, however, only modestly augments cardiac output and coronary blood flow and is unable to provide total circulatory support when hemodynamic collapse occurs [20]. Although the IABP restored epicardial perfusion in animal models, it had little effect on microvascular flow in the setting of acute myocardial infarction [21]. Furthermore, the IABP requires a certain level of left ventricular function. In addition, it has not been independently associated with improved cardiac function or able to reverse cardiogenic shock and provide a survival benefit [22–24].

Hemodynamic effects of the intra-aortic balloon pump

The effects of the IABP include decreases in heart rate, left ventricular end-diastolic pressure, mean left atrial pressure, afterload, and myocardial oxygen consumption by at least 20% to 30% [25]. The IABP also modestly increases coronary perfusion pressure and decreases the right atrial pressure, pulmonary artery pressure, and pulmonary vascular resistance. No significant changes in the mean aortic pressure have been observed, however, and it only modestly augments cardiac output [26]. The IABP is also dependent on an intrinsic cardiac rhythm. Furthermore, it is ineffective in patients in cardiac arrest or in patients who have severe left ventricular dysfunction.

TandemHeart

The TandemHeart percutaneous LVAD (Fig. 1) is a left atrial-to-femoral bypass system that can provide rapid short-term circulatory support with resolution of pulmonary edema and deranged metabolism in patients who have cardiogenic shock [27]. In an animal model of acute myocardial infarction and cardiogenic shock, the left atrial-to-femoral artery bypass assist device restored endocardial (microvascular) and epicardial blood flow to baseline [26] and resulted in a substantial reduction in the infarct size [28]. The TandemHeart has advantages over earlier LVADs because it can be implanted percutaneously and provides rapid hemodynamic support regardless of the native heart rhythm.

The TandemHeart has been used in a variety of situations, including in high-risk PCI patients, in acute myocardial infarction patients in cardiogenic shock, and in decompensated heart failure with myocarditis. The TandemHeart has also been used in cardiac surgery patients to preoperatively unload the left ventricle and provide mechanical circulatory support during the perioperative and postoperative period until cardiac function sufficiently recovers or until an LVAD can be surgically implanted for long-term hemodynamic support.

There are three subsystems that make up the TandemHeart system. The first subsystem is a

Table 1
Percutaneous ventricular assist devices

Device	Pump	Speed (rpm)	Duration	Cardiac support	Anticoagulation	Motor
TandemHeart	Centrifugal	3000–7500	Up to 14 d	Up to 4 L/min	Required	Rotor powered by electromagnetic coupling
Impella Recover LP 2.5 System	Axial	Up to 50,000	Up to 5 d	Up to 2.5 L/min	Required	Integrated electric motor

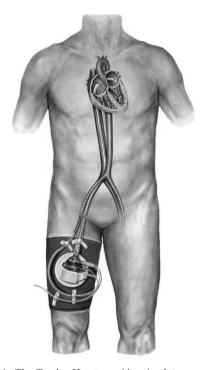

Fig. 1. The TandemHeart provides circulatory support by continuously withdrawing oxygenated blood from the left atrium by way of a transseptal cannula placed in the femoral vein. The pump then returns blood by way of the femoral artery. The hemodynamic effects of the TandemHeart include an increase in cardiac output and blood pressure and a decrease in afterload and pre-load, thus decreasing myocardial oxygen demand. (Courtesy of CardiacAssist, Pittsburgh, Pennsylvania.)

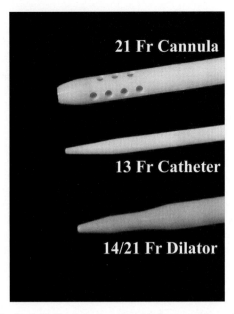

Fig. 2. A 21 F venous transseptal inflow cannula made of polyurethane contains a large end hole and 14 side holes to allow for aspiration of the oxygenated blood from the left atrium. A two-stage (14/21 F) dilator is used to dilate the transseptal puncture after a 0.035-inch pigtail guidewire is inserted into the left atrium. The obturator is tapered at its tip to allow for easy insertion into the left atrium. (Courtesy of CardiacAssist, Pittsburgh, Pennsylvania.)

21 F venous transseptal inflow cannula that is made of polyurethane (Fig. 2). This cannula has a curved design at its end to facilitate ideal tip placement in the left atrium and contains a large end hole at its distal tip and 14 side holes to aspirate oxygenated blood from the left atrium. The obturator is tapered at its tip to allow for easy insertion into the left atrium. The cannula is attached to a continuous-flow centrifugal blood pump. This compact pump contains a hydrodynamic fluid bearing to support a six-bladed rotating impeller that provides up to 4 L/min of pump flow (Fig. 3). Power is supplied by a direct current brushless electromagnetic motor that operates at a range of 3000 to 7500 rpm. There are generous gaps between the impella and the housing which permits blood to flow freely with low friction, thereby limiting the generation of heat, hemolysis, and thromboembolism [29]. Blood is then delivered

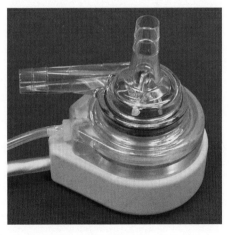

Fig. 3. The continuous-flow centrifugal blood pump contains a hydrodynamic fluid bearing to support a six-bladed rotating impeller that provides up to 4 L/min of pump flow. (Courtesy of CardiacAssist, Pittsburgh, Pennsylvania.)

from the pump to the femoral artery with an arterial perfusion catheter. This catheter ranges from 15 to 17 F and pumps blood from the left atrium to the right femoral artery. Alternatively, two 12 F arterial perfusion catheters pump blood into the right and left femoral arteries.

The pump is driven by the external microprocessor-based controller. A constant 10 mL/h flow of saline with unfractionated heparin is infused into the pump to provide (1) fluid bearing for the rotor, (2) local anticoagulation for the pump chamber to prevent the formation of thrombus, (3) systemic lubrication, and (4) cooling of the unit (Fig. 4). A pressure transducer monitors the infusion pressure and identifies any disruption in the infusion line. An in-line air bubble detector monitors for the presence of air in the infusion line.

Contraindications

Because adequate left atrial pressures are required for sufficient pumping, the TandemHeart is contraindicated in patients who have predominant right ventricular failure [27]. Patients who have a ventricular septal defect are not good candidates for the TandemHeart because of the risk of hypoxemia due to right-to-left shunting.

Because the left ventricle can become distended in the setting of severe left ventricular dysfunction and impedes subendocardial perfusion, aortic insufficiency is another contraindication to the TandemHeart. The TandemHeart can induce critical limb ischemia in patients who have severe peripheral vascular disease.

Implantation

The TandemHeart is implanted in the cardiac catheterization laboratory. Under fluoroscopic guidance, a transseptal puncture with the Brockenbrough needle is inserted through a Mullins sheath into the superior vena cava to obtain access from the right atrium into the left atrium (Fig. 5). A two-stage (14/21 F) dilator is used to dilate the transseptal puncture after a 0.035-inch pigtail guidewire is inserted into the left atrium. Subsequently, the transseptal cannula is inserted into the right femoral vein, advanced over the guidewire toward the right atrium, and placed into the left atrium. All of the side holes of the transseptal cannula are required to be completely

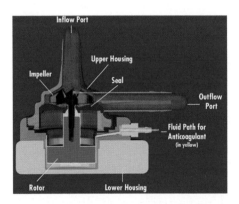

Fig. 4. Cutaway section of TandemHeart. The Tandem-Heart has a dual-chamber pump. The upper housing provides a conduit for inflow and outflow of blood. The lower housing provides communication with the controller, the ability to rotate the impeller, and a fluid path for a constant 10 mL/h flow of saline with unfractionated heparin, which is infused into the pump to provide (1) fluid bearing for the rotor, (2) local anticoagulation for the pump chamber to prevent the formation of thrombus, (3) systemic lubrication, and (4) cooling of the unit. (Courtesy of CardiacAssist, Pittsburgh, Pennsylvania.)

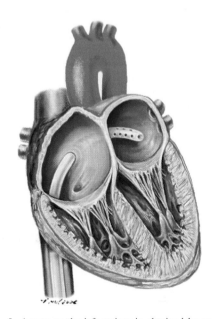

Fig. 5. Access to the left atrium is obtained by way of standard transseptal techniques. Catheter exchanges are made with the valvuloplasty wire. The septum is dilated with a two-stage dilator. Next, the cannula is placed into the left atrium while ensuring all drainage holes are in the left atrium (last 2.5 cm of the cannula). (Courtesy of CardiacAssist, Pittsburgh, Pennsylvania.)

positioned in the left atrium to avoid right-to-left shunting. After the position of the cannula is confirmed by angiography and echocardiography, the guidewire and obturator are removed. The cannula is then sutured to the skin over the thigh and cross-clamped with a vascular clamp.

Because of the risk of critical limb ischemia in patients who have severe peripheral vascular disease, an iliofemoral angiogram before implantation of the arterial perfusion catheter is crucial. The tip of the arterial outflow cannula is advanced to the level of the aortic bifurcation over a guidewire after access in the right femoral artery is obtained. After the air is purged from the extracorporeal system, the transseptal cannula is attached to the inflow port of the centrifugal blood pump in the standard wet-to-wet fashion with 3/8 inch. Tygon tubing. The power supply for the TandemHeart is subsequently connected to the microprocessor-based controller (Fig. 6). With skilled and experienced operators, the entire insertion, assembly, and mechanical circulatory support can be accomplished in 30 minutes or less. Because of the risk of thromboembolic complications, systemic anticoagulation with unfractionated heparin to maintain an activated clotting time of 400 seconds during insertion and 200 seconds during support is mandatory. The TandemHeart has been used for up to 14 days [5].

Explantation

When the TandemHeart is ready to be discontinued, the percutaneous arterial and venous cannulas can easily be removed percutaneously after the heparin drip and pump are turned off. When the activated clotting time is low enough to allow for safe removal of the arterial cannula, hemostasis is obtained with manual compression of the puncture site. A small iatrogenic atrial septal defect is left after the explantation of the transseptal cannula, which resolves after 4 to 6 weeks or has no clinically significant left-to-right shunt [28]. A bubble study demonstrated no echocardiographic evidence of a residual atrial septal defect after removal of the transseptal cannula [5].

Hemodynamic effects

The TandemHeart provides circulatory support by diverting oxygenated blood from the left atrium into systemic circulation, which increases cardiac output and blood pressure and decreases afterload and preload, thus decreasing myocardial oxygen demand. The increase in mean arterial pressure may optimize the supply and demand of oxygen in the myocardium at risk and increase tissue perfusion at the coronary and peripheral level [27]. This increase in tissue perfusion leads to the reversal of metabolic acidosis and a decrease in serum lactate levels in patients who have cardiogenic shock. In addition, Doppler flow studies of the carotid vasculature demonstrate augmentation of carotid artery flow during diastole (Fig. 7).

Potential complications

The transseptal puncture required for the TandemHeart is a potential source of complications (Box 1). Inadvertent puncture of the aortic root, coronary sinus, or posterior free wall of the right atrium can lead to disastrous complications

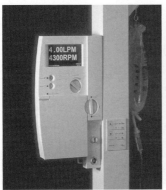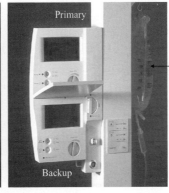

Fig. 6. TandemHeart microprocessor-based controller has a primary and backup control unit to reduce the need for back-up equipment. (Courtesy of CardiacAssist, Pittsburgh, Pennsylvania.)

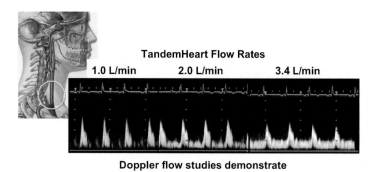

TandemHeart Flow Rates

1.0 L/min   2.0 L/min   3.4 L/min

**Doppler flow studies demonstrate
diastolic augmentation**

Fig. 7. Carotid artery flow at varying TandemHeart rpm. Doppler flow studies of the carotid vasculature demonstrate augmentation of carotid artery flow during diastole. (Courtesy of CardiacAssist, Pittsburgh, Pennsylvania.)

including death. Thromboembolism can be another potential source of complication. Cerebral thromboembolism occurred in a patient who formed thrombus at the edge of a large ventricular septal defect and at the site of the left atrial puncture despite anticoagulation with unfractionated heparin [27]. Because unfractionated heparin is needed to achieve a high activated clotting time, bleeding, especially from the groin, can occur with the TandemHeart. Systemic hypothermia can occur when contact of the system circuit with room temperature leads to the cooling of the blood flowing through the pump [30]. Accidental dislodgement of the arterial cannula has led to acute decompensation and death from cardiogenic shock [27]. Local infections, bacteremia, and sepsis are potential complications with any implantable device.

Potential applications

In addition to providing hemodynamic support in patients who have cardiogenic shock and in high-risk PCI patients, potential applications for the TandemHeart include high-risk aortic

valvuloplasty, percutaneous aortic valve replacement, and functioning as a percutaneous right ventricular assist device for right heart failure (Fig. 8). A high-risk patient underwent PCI for ostial left main coronary artery stenosis (Fig. 9), ostial right coronary artery stenosis (Fig. 10), and aortic valvuloplasty for critical aortic stenosis (aortic valve area of 0.53 cm^2) with the support of the TandemHeart (Fig. 11) [30].

Impella CardioSystems

The Impella Recover LP 2.5 System (Fig. 12) is one of four percutaneous or minimally invasive ventricular unloading catheters manufactured by

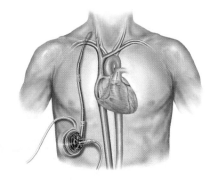

Fig. 8. In addition to providing hemodynamic support in patients who have cardiogenic shock and in high-risk PCI patients, potential applications for the Tandem-Heart include functioning as a percutaneous right ventricular assist device for right heart failure. The 21 F venous transseptal inflow cannula aspirates oxygenated blood from the right atrium. Blood is then delivered from the pump to the pulmonary artery with an arterial perfusion catheter. (Courtesy of CardiacAssist, Pittsburgh, Pennsylvania.)

Box 1. Potential complications of the TandemHeart

Puncture of aortic root, coronary sinus, or posterior free wall of right atrium
Thromboembolism
Systemic hypothermia
Cannula dislodgement
Bleeding
Infection

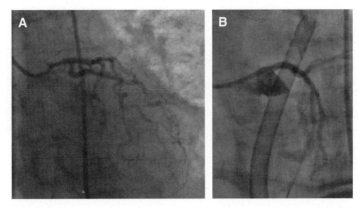

Fig. 9. The ostial left main coronary artery showing severe stenosis (*A*). An excellent angiographic result was obtained after stenting with a 3.0 × 8 mm Cypher (Cordis, Johnson and Johnson Corp.; Miami, Florida) drug-eluting stent (*B*).

Impella CardioSystems. These devices have been used in Europe to provide rapid and short-term hemodynamic support in patients who have acute heart failure, acute myocardial infarction, PCI, and during and after cardiac surgery (especially for postcardiotomy low cardiac output syndrome) by aspirating blood from the left ventricle and expelling it to the ascending aorta. The Impella Recover LP 2.5 System implements a miniaturized rotary blood pump that provides circulatory assist in acute myocardial infarction, cardiogenic shock or low-output states, or during high-risk PCI for up to 5 days.

The intracardiac axial flow pump contains a rotor that is driven by an electrical motor and has an inflow cannula. The left ventricular pump can provide up to 2.5 L/min of cardiac output, depending on the speed of the rotor (which can operate at a maximum of 50,000 rpm), and the difference between aortic blood pressure and left ventricular pressure. Located in the front of the rotor is a differential pressure sensor that monitors this difference in pressure (Fig. 13). The appropriate position of the flow pump can be confirmed by the pressure difference between the aorta and left ventricle. The system has a catheter coming from the patient that connects to a mobile console that permits the management of the rotational speed of the pump and displays of the differences of pressure between the inflow and outflow (Fig. 14). The Impella pump is continuously purged with a glucose solution (10%) that is drawn into a 50-mL syringe with heparin (2500 IU) (Fig. 15). The purge flow rates normally range from 2 to 6 mL/h to continuously rinse and prevent thrombus formation in the pump.

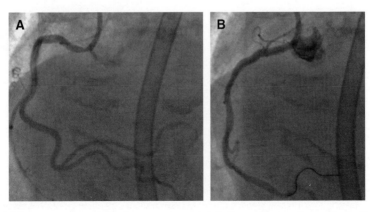

Fig. 10. The ostial right coronary artery showing severe stenosis (*A*). An excellent angiographic result was obtained after stenting with a 3.0 × 13 mm Cypher (Cordis, Johnson and Johnson Corp.; Miami, Florida) drug-eluting stent (*B*).

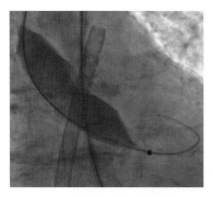

Fig. 11. The aortic valve gradient was 75 mm Hg and the aortic valve area was 0.53 cm^2. After crossing the aortic valve with a 6 F multipurpose catheter and standard glidewire (Boston Scientific, Natick, Massachusetts) and exchanging the glidewire with a stiff Amplatz (Cook, Bloomington, Indiana) 260-cm wire, a 5.0 × 20 mm Zmed-II valvuloplasty balloon (Numed, Hopkinton, New York) was inflated twice. The final gradient across the aortic valve was 16 to 20 mm Hg and the aortic valve area was 0.8 cm^2.

Contraindications

In addition to severe peripheral vascular disease, the Impella Recover LP 2.5 System is contraindicated in patients who have mechanical aortic valves or heavily calcified aortic valves.

Implantation

The Impella Recover LP 2.5 System, which is 4 mm in diameter (12 F), is mounted on a 9 F pigtail catheter and inserted percutaneously in the

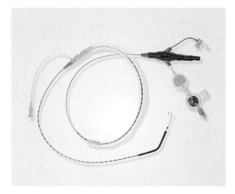

Fig. 12. The Impella Recover LP 2.5 System is an LVAD that provides hemodynamic support in patients that can be inserted percutaneously. The pigtail tip is inserted into the left ventricle to withdraw blood into the aorta. (Courtesy of Impella CardioSystems, Aachen, Germany.)

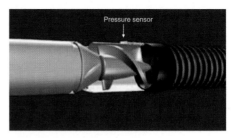

Fig. 13. The intracardiac axial flow pump contains a rotor that is driven by an electrical motor and has an inflow cannula. Blood is drawn in at the tip of the cannula and is expelled at the sides upstream from the motor into the aorta. A differential pressure sensor measures the difference in pressure between the inflow and outflow of the pump. (Courtesy of Impella CardioSystems, Aachen, Germany.)

cardiac catheterization laboratory into the femoral artery over a guidewire through a peel-away introducer with a removable hemostatic valve (Fig. 16). An advantage of the Impella over the TandemHeart is that there is no need for a transseptal puncture and no extracorporeal blood. The inflow cannula miniaturized pump is inserted through the aortic valve under fluoroscopic guidance into the left ventricle to pump blood from the left ventricle into the ascending aorta (Fig. 17) [31]. If the patient also has an IABP on the

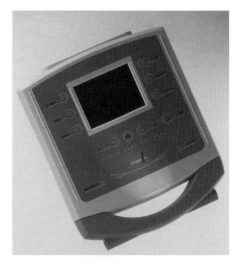

Fig. 14. The mobile console permits the management of the rotational speed of the pump and displays of the differences of pressure between the inflow and outflow. It provides 60 minutes of battery time and nine flow settings. (Courtesy of Impella CardioSystems, Aachen, Germany.)

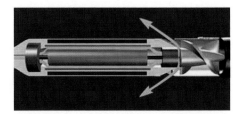

Fig. 15. The Impella motor is continuously purged with a glucose solution (10%) that is drawn into a 50-mL syringe with heparin (2500 IU) The purge flow rates normally range from 2 to 6 mL/h to continuously rinse and prevent thrombus formation in the pump. (Courtesy of Impella CardioSystems, Aachen, Germany.)

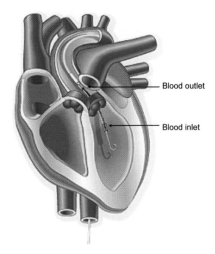

Fig. 17. The Impella is placed across the aortic valve allowing the pump to aspirate blood from the left ventricle and expel it to the ascending aorta. The Impella implements a miniaturized rotary blood pump that provides circulatory assist in acute myocardial infarction, cardiogenic shock, low-output states, or during high-risk PCI for up to 5 days. (Courtesy of Impella CardioSystems, Aachen, Germany.)

contralateral groin, it can be put on standby as the Impella pump is being positioned. Continuous anticoagulation with heparin to maintain the activated clotting time above 160 seconds is required to minimize thromboembolism while the pump is in use.

Hemodynamics effects

The Impella pump rapidly unloads the left ventricle by delivering blood into the ascending

aorta. In an animal model, the Impella pump reduced myocardial oxygen consumption during ischemia and reperfusion, leading to a reduced infarct size [32]. Patients who have cardiogenic shock treated with the Impella pump system had improvements in cardiac output and mean blood pressure and a reduction in pulmonary capillary wedge pressure [31]. Compared with the IABP, the Impella pump improved cardiac and systemic hemodynamics during acute mitral regurgitation in an animal model [33]. No significant increase in aortic regurgitation was observed with intracardiac echocardiography when the catheter was through the aortic valve [34].

The average pressure-volume loops demonstrate a reduction in the left ventricular end-diastolic pressure (18–11 mm Hg), end-diastolic volume (345–321 mL), and stroke volume (94–76 mL) [34].

Potential complications

Meyns and colleagues [31] reported the loss of the sensor signal in three patients, which did not affect pump function. Similar to the TandemHeart, an iliofemoral angiogram before sheath insertion is indicated because of the risk of critical limb ischemia in patients who have severe peripheral

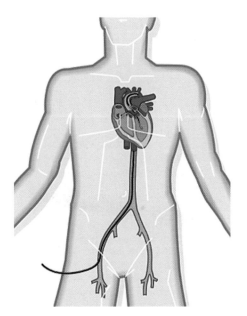

Fig. 16. The Impella pump, which is 4 mm in diameter (12 F), is mounted on a 9 F pigtail catheter and inserted percutaneously in the cardiac catheterization laboratory into the femoral artery over a guidewire through a peel-away introducer with a removable hemostatic valve. (Courtesy of Impella CardioSystems, Aachen, Germany.)

vascular disease. No patients have required treatment for hemolysis when treated with the Impella Recover LP 2.5 System. Displacement of the pump back into the aorta can also occur, but the addition of the pigtail catheter tip minimizes displacement potential. Similar to the TandemHeart, the percutaneous blood cannulae pose the inherent risk of infectious complications in the form of local infections, bacteremia, and sepsis.

Summary

Patients undergoing PCI who have severely compromised left ventricular systolic function and complex coronary lesions including multivessel disease, left main disease, or bypass graft disease are at higher risk of adverse outcomes from hemodynamic collapse. The TandemHeart percutaneous LVAD and the Impella Recover LP 2.5 System can provide short-term hemodynamic stability in patients who require hemodynamic support in a variety of settings. Both devices provide more ventricular support than the IABP and can be implanted rapidly and percutaneously in a prophylactic or emergency setting. Identification of those who are at high risk for severe hemodynamic compromise and most likely to benefit from mechanical circulatory support is crucial to derive the greatest benefit from this modality. Multicenter randomized clinical trials are needed to clearly define the role of these two devices in providing circulatory support in a variety of clinical settings.

References

[1] Black A, Cortina R, Bossi I, et al. Unprotected left main coronary artery stenting: correlates of midterm survival and impact of patient selection. J Am Coll Cardiol 2001;37:832–8.

[2] Ellis SG, Tamai H, Nobuyoshi M, et al. Contemporary percutaneous treatment of unprotected left main coronary stenoses: initial results from a multicenter registry analysis 1994–1996. Circulation 1997; 96:3867–72.

[3] Kosuga K, Tamai H, Ueda K, et al. Initial and long-term results of angioplasty in unprotected left main coronary artery. Am J Cardiol 1999;83:32–7.

[4] Kar B, Butkevich A, Civitello AB, et al. Hemodynamic support with a percutaneous left ventricular assist device. Tex Heart Inst J 2004;31:84–6.

[5] Vranckx P, Foley DP, de Feijter PJ, et al. Effective use of the TandemHeart during high-risk percutaneous coronary intervention. Int J Cardiovasc Intervent 2003;5:35–9.

[6] Aragon J, Lee MS, Kar S, et al. Percutaneous left ventricular assist device: "TandemHeart" for high-risk coronary intervention. Catheter Cardiovasc Interv 2005;65:346–52.

[7] Becker RC, Gore JM, Lambrew C, et al. A composite view of cardiac rupture in the United States National Registry of Myocardial Infarction. J Am Coll Cardiol 1996;27:1321–6.

[8] Scheidt S, Wilner G, Mueller H, et al. Intra-aortic balloon counterpulsation in cardiogenic shock: report of a co-operative clinical trial. N Engl J Med 1973;288:979–84.

[9] DeWood MA, Notske RN, Hensley GR, et al. Intra-aortic balloon counterpulsation with and without reperfusion for myocardial infarction shock. Circulation 1980;61:1105–12.

[10] Catinella FP, Cuningham JN, Glassman E, et al. Left atrium-to-femoral artery bypass: effectiveness in reduction of acute experimental myocardial infarction. J Thorac Cardiovasc Surg 1983;86:887–96.

[11] Grossi EA, Krieger KH, Cunningham JN, et al. Time course of effective interventional left heart assist for limitation of evolving myocardial infarction. J Thorac Cardiovasc Surg 1986;91:624–9.

[12] Laschinger JC, Grossi EA, Cunningham JN Jr, et al. Adjunctive left ventricular unloading during myocardial reperfusion plays a major role in minimizing myocardial infarct size. J Thorac Cardiovasc Surg 1985;90:80–5.

[13] Frazier OH, Rose EA, Macmanus Q, et al. Multicenter clinical evaluation of the HeartMate 1000 IP left ventricular assist device. Ann Thorac Surg 1992;53: 1080–90.

[14] Chen JM, DeRose JJ, Slater JP. Improved survival rates support LVAD implantation early after myocardial infarction. J Am Coll Cardiol 1999;33: 1903–8.

[15] Vogel RA, Shawl F, Tommaso C, et al. Initial report of the national registry of elective cardiopulmonary bypass supported coronary angioplasty. J Am Coll Cardiol 1990;15:23–9.

[16] Shawl F, Domanski MJ, Wish MH, et al. Percutaneous cardiopulmonary bypass support in the catheterization laboratory: technique and complications. Am Heart J 1990;120:195–203.

[17] Kaul U, Sahay S, Bahl VK, et al. Coronary angioplasty in high-risk patients: comparison of elective intraaortic balloon pump and percutaneous cardiopulmonary bypass support-a randomized study. J Interv Cardiol 1995;8:199–205.

[18] Scholz KH, Dubois-Rande JL, Urban P, et al. Clinical experience with the percutaneous hemopump during high-risk coronary angioplasty. Am J Cardiol 1998;82:1107–10.

[19] Kantrowitz A, Tjonneland S, Freed PS, et al. Initial clinical experience with intraaortic balloon pumping in cardiogenic shock. JAMA 1968;203:113–8.

[20] Nanas JN, Moulopoulos SD. Counterpulsation: historical background, technical improvements, he-

modynamic and metabolic effects. Cardiology 1994; 84:156–67.

[21] Hata M, Shiono M, Orime Y, et al. Coronary microcirculation during left heart bypass with a centrifugal pump. Artif Organs 1996;20:678–80.

[22] Stone GW, Marsalese D, Brodie BR, et al. A prospective, randomized evaluation of prophylactic intraaortic balloon counterpulsation in high risk patients with acute myocardial infarction treated with primary angioplasty. Second Primary Angioplasty in Myocardial Infarction (PAMI-II) Trial Investigators. J Am Coll Cardiol 1997;29:1459–67.

[23] Berger PB, Holmes DR Jr, Stebbins AL, et al. Impact of an aggressive invasive catheterization and revascularization strategy on mortality in patients with cardiogenic shock in the Global Utilization of Streptokinase and Tissue Plasminogen Activator for Occluded Coronary Arteries (GUSTO-1) trial. Circulation 1997;96:122–7.

[24] Pae W, Pierce W. Temporary left ventricular assistance in acute myocardial infarction and cardiogenic shock. Chest 1981;79:692–5.

[25] Mahaffey KW, Kruse KR, Ohman EM. Perspectives on the use of intra-aortic balloon counterpulsation in the 1990s. In: Topol EJ, editor. Textbook of interventional cardiology. (Update 21). Philadelphia: WB Saunders; 1996. p. 303–21.

[26] Mulukutla SR, Pacella JJ, Cohen HA. Contemporary cardiology: cardiogenic shock: diagnosis and treatment. Totowa (NJ): Humana Press; 2002. p. 303–24.

[27] Thiele H, Lauer B, Hambrecht R, et al. Reversal of cardiogenic shock by percutaneous left atrial-to-femoral atrial bypass assistance. Circulation 2001; 104:2917–22.

[28] Fonger JD, Zhou Y, Matsuura H, et al. Enhanced preservation of acutely ischemic myocardium with transseptal left ventricular assist. Ann Thorac Surg 1994;57:570–5.

[29] Lemos PA, Cummins P, Lee CH, et al. Usefulness of percutaneous left ventricular assistance to support high-risk percutaneous coronary interventions. Am J Cardiol 2003;91:479–81.

[30] Makkar RR, Aragon J, Soleimani T, et al. Ostial left main stenosis, ostial right coronary stenosis and aortic valvuloplasty performed with the support of the TandemHeart percutaneous left ventricular assist device. Available at: http://www.tctmd.com. Accessed February 14, 2005.

[31] Meyns B, Dens J, Sergeant P, et al. Initial experiences with the Impella-device in patients with cardiogenic shock. Thorac Cardio Surg 2003;51:1–6.

[32] Meyns B, Stolinski J, Leunens V, et al. Left ventricular support by catheter-mounted axial flow pump reduces infarct size. J Am Coll Cardiol 2003;41: 1087–95.

[33] Reesink K, Dekker A, van der Nagel T, et al. New Impella intracardiac minipump supports the acutely failing left heart significantly more effective than intra aortic balloon pumping [abstract]. J Am Coll Cardiol 2003;41:215A.

[34] Valgimigli M, Steendijk P, Sianos G, et al. Left ventricular unloading and concomitant total cardiac output increase by the use of percutaneous Impella Recover LP 2.5 assist device during high-risk coronary intervention. Cathet Cardiovasc Interv 2005;65:263–7.

Vascular Closure Devices

Michael C. Kim, MD

*Cardiac Catheterization Laboratory, The Mount Sinai School of Medicine, 5 East 98th Street,
3rd Floor, New York, NY 10029, USA*

As the number of femoral artery catheterizations continues to increase over the next decade to more than 9 million, the importance of quick, efficient, and effective vascular closure techniques cannot be overemphasized. Vascular access complications remain the leading source of morbidity, cost, and legal ramifications after a cardiac catheterization, with or without percutaneous coronary intervention (PCI) [1]. Any experienced interventional cardiologist knows the importance of vascular access and hemostasis; many patients remember only the pain of entering and closing the artery. Patients who return for a repeat catheterization often do not worry about the actual procedure, but are concerned about the length of time that they are required to remain in bed afterward.

Vascular complications—reported to be as high as 14%—with PCI lead to increased hospital length of stay and hospital costs [2]. Vascular closure devices (VCDs) were introduced in 1995 to decrease complications and the time to hemostasis and ambulation. Although the frequency of complications with VCDs is debatable, the VCD market has become a greater than $500 million industry because of advances in patient comfort and physician efficiency [3].

In 1953, Dr. Sven-Ivar Seldinger [4], a radiologist from Sweden, published his landmark paper that detailed the Seldinger percutaneous technique for obtaining femoral artery access. In that paper, he described the technique of manual compression (MC), which has been the gold standard for vascular access hemostasis for more than 50 years. The access site should be held with direct pressure for 20 to 30 minutes followed by overnight bed rest. Only over the last decade has this technique been challenged with the introduction of VCDs as the numbers of PCIs increased and the antiplatelet and anticoagulation regimens became more complicated.

This article summarizes the VCD technologies that are available to physicians who perform percutaneous catheter-based procedures.

Patches

Vascular closure patches still require MC. It is a possible means of decreasing time to hemostasis and time to ambulation. This is helpful to improve throughput in the laboratory at a cost that is less than a VCD; however, no randomized clinical trial has comparing the efficacy of these patches with MC or VCDs. The major advantage of patches over VCDs is a lower purchasing cost and less hardware in the patient.

Syvek Patch

The Syvek Patch (Marine Polymer Technologies, Inc., Danvers, Massachusetts) is based on the ability of poly-N-acetylglucosamine (pGIcNAc) to promote vasoconstriction, red blood cell agglutination, and platelet activation for fibrin clot formation. Studies have shown that pGIcNAc helps to promote vasoconstriction by way of endothelin-1 activation. Animal models also demonstrated red blood cell agglutination when a patch laced with pGIcNAc was placed on an open wound. Its mechanism of action is unknown. Furthermore, studies demonstrated the activation of platelets when in contact with pGIcNAc, which leads to rapid fibrinogen cross-linking and platelet aggregation.

Several small trials showed effective hemostasis using the Syvek Patch when applied for 10 minutes

E-mail address: michael.kim@msnyuhealth.org

cardiology.theclinics.com

or less. One study showed safety in discharging patients after 2 hours when using the patch [5]. The largest study, by Nader and colleagues [6], looked at 1000 consecutive patients who used the Syvek Patch. The 636 diagnostic procedures required 10 minutes of compression and the 364 PCI procedures required 20 minutes of patch compression. This observational study showed a major complication rate of 0.1% (pseudoaneurysm in the PCI group), and a minor complication of 1.3% (mostly small hematomas and nuisance bleeds).

Scion Clo-Sur P.A.D.

The Clo-Sur P.A.D. (Scion Cardiovascular, Miami, Florida) is a soft, nonwoven hydrophilic wound dressing that contains a naturally occurring biopolymer (polyprolate acetate). This biopolymer is cationically charged, and it is theorized that the positive ionic charges interact with the negatively charged red blood cells and platelets, and result in the acceleration of a naturally forming fibrin and platelet clot. It has been approved by the Food and Drug Administration (FDA) for management in bleeding wounds. A single center looked at 122 patients (40 PCIs) who used the Clo-Sur P.A.D. for at least 10 minutes; most ambulated within 2 hours [7]. There were no major complications in the PCI group and 2 patients in the diagnostic catheterization group developed a pseudoaneurysm that was diagnosed 4 days after the procedure.

Chito-Seal pad

The Chito-Seal pad (Abbott Vascular Devices, Redwood City, California) is similar to the Clo-Sur P.A.D. This pad is approved by the FDA for the management of bleeding wounds, including vascular access sites. It is coated with Abbott's proprietary chitosan gel, a powerful hemostatic agent. Chitosan gel is twice as chemically active as chitin, the biopolymer from which it is derived. When placed over a bleeding wound, it becomes a cell-binding agent that consists of positively charged chitosan molecules that attract negatively charged red blood cells and platelets; it is designed to accelerate natural clot formation.

Only one study has compared different patches. Fisher and colleagues [8] used a coagulopathic swine spleen-bleeding model to compare the Syvek Patch with the Clo-Sur P.A.D. and the Chito-Seal pad. The Syvek Patch produced in vitro red blood cell aggregation and reduced the time to in vitro fibrin clot formation using platelet-rich plasma samples in 100% of cases compared with 50% of cases when using a dry gauze. The Clo-Sur P.A.D. achieved hemostasis in no cases, whereas the Chito-Seal pad achieved hemostasis in only 25% of cases.

D-Stat products

D-Stat products (Vascular Solutions, Minneapolis, Minnesota) are a family of topical hemostats that are coated with thrombin, and thereby, stimulate the production of fibrinogen, which activates fibrin hemostasis. Products include a foam pad, gel, bandage, radial pressure device, and a clamp accessory device. No randomized clinical trials have been published to confirm their efficacy over standard compression devices or MC.

Suture-mediated closure devices

Suture-mediated closure devices have distinct advantages and disadvantages. Devices that can deliver a U-stitch at the arteriotomy site have a long history of effective hemostasis; vascular surgeons have been using the technique for decades in the operating room. The original Sones' technique of brachial artery access for diagnostic cardiac catheterization used a cut-down to access the artery and manual sutures to close the brachial artery access site. Additionally, immediate reaccess at the femoral artery site can be performed using this technique, because there are no concerns of placing a new sheath over the old site or suture. Compare that with devices that use collagen/thrombin plugs at the site where a new sheath could embolize the plug into the femoral artery and produce thrombosis of the leg or disrupt the plug in the tissue tract, which leads to bleeding at the previous arteriotomy site. Vascular surgeons have reported a diminished inflammatory response to suture-mediated closure techniques at the tissue tract site [9]; the clinical relevance of this is unknown.

Perclose

The Perclose Prostar (Abbott Vascular Devices) device was introduced in 1994 as the first suture-mediated device to be approved by the FDA. Using a braided polyester suture, the Prostar can close 6.5F to 8F access sites. It is designed to provide complete tissue apposition that results in primary healing. Initial studies showed a reduced time to hemostasis, ambulation, and discharge in diagnostic femoral artery catheterization compared with MC.

Each case requires a femoral angiogram to ensure proper sheath placement in the common femoral artery and to rule out significant peripheral vascular disease (PVD). The Perclose device requires five successful steps for hemostasis. First, one must position the device into the femoral artery. When the device is placed ideally in the femoral artery, blood will be seen through the marker lumen. The foot pedals are deployed inside the arteries and the device is pulled until pressure is felt. Second, the needles are deployed. Third, the plunger must be removed, which allows the suture to be retrieved. Next, the suture is harvested and must be knotted. The fifth and final step is knot advancement of the suture until it is placed at the femoral arteriotomy site. One tests for hemostasis by asking the patient to cough, and the suture is cut above the artery within the tissue tract.

The Prostar was never able to capture a large market share because of the complexity of deploying the device. The needle and suture was placed into the artery by the device but it had to be retrieved within the tissue tract manually and then knotted using a separate manual device that was included in the Prostar package. The end result was a complicated and time-consuming device that led to many points at which error could be introduced. The Prostar XL is still available if one needs to close a 8.5F to 10F access site.

In 1997, the Perclose Closer was introduced as a more user-friendly suture-mediated closure device. Additionally, studies showed that it was an effective alternative to MC in anticoagulated patients who were undergoing PCI. This device was a smaller 6F device where the needle deployment occurs from outside the femoral artery; this allows the device to capture the suture automatically by the device. The operator then knots the suture using the manual knot-tying device that is provided. Although this advance allowed for a quicker deployment of the device, it was still cumbersome because of the time needed to produce a knot and then deploy it to the arteriotomy site.

In 2002, The Perclose A-T (Auto-Tie) was introduced. This marked a major step in suture-mediated closure because time to closure was reduced significantly. The Perclose A-T produces a pretied knot that obviates the need for the manual knot-tying device. This step was considered the most technically demanding and the most time consuming. The auto-tie feature decreased the procedure time and led to a decrease in unsuccessful deployments. Additionally, the auto-tie function allows for true single-operator deployment.

In 2004, the most recent Perclose model, called the Proglide, was introduced. The Proglide uses a polypropylene monofilament suture in place of the polyester braided suture that was used in previous models. This monofilament suture reportedly increases knotted tensile strength, provides easier knot delivery because the material is more slippery, and is designed to provide less inflammatory response compared with a braided suture. The Proglide maintains the automated knot tying with a pretied, heat-set knot and adds a quick-cut mechanism that eliminates the need for extra sharps or a sterile scissor (Fig. 1).

The Perclose system represents approximately 35% to 40% of the VCD market. It is quick, reliable, and effective in producing hemostasis in diagnostic interventional cases that use the femoral artery. It can be deployed by a single operator and allows for immediate reaccess. Because the catheter remains in the femoral artery until it is removed, it allows for reintroduction of a wire and sheath into the artery if the device fails to deploy the needles or suture appropriately. Because the risk for a vascular complication is greatest when a VCD fails, this advantage cannot be overemphasized. Complications include infection, laceration of the artery by the foot pedals, and posterior wall partial dissection by the foot pedal that may lead to abrupt or subacute femoral artery closure or thrombosis that is due to inadvertent knotting of the posterior dissection plane to the anterior femoral arteriotomy site by way of the sutures. Early trials with the Prostar version showed a 90% successful deployment rate with a minor vascular complication rate of 5% and a major complication rate of 3% to 4% [10].

X-Site suture closure device

The X-Site (Datascope Corp., Montvale, New Jersey) suture-mediated closure device is an alternative to Perclose. Using a braided polyester suture, the X-Site device is able to deploy the needles and suture through the femoral artery without the use of foot pedals, which decreases the possibility of any intra-arterial trauma. Because there is no auto-tie mechanism in the device, however, it will not be available until 2007.

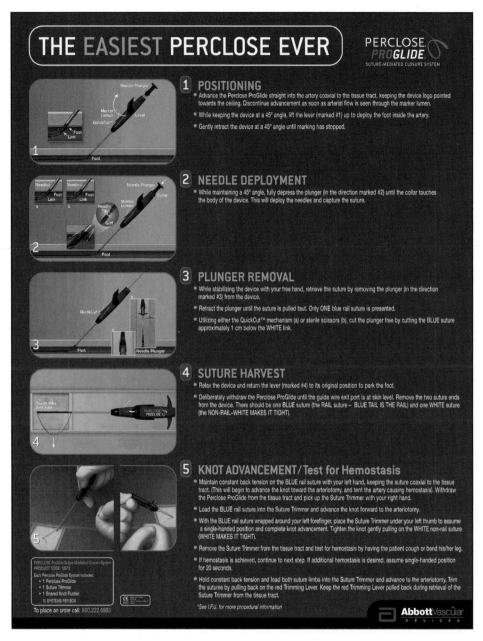

Fig. 1. Perclose Proglide deployment. Five-step deployment process for suture-mediated closure. (Courtesy of Abbott Vascular, Redwood City, CA.)

The randomized trial that led to FDA approval of the device showed a striking decrease in vascular complications compared with MC. The Rapid Ambulation to Closure trial randomized 250 patients who underwent diagnostic or PCI procedures to the X-Site device or MC. There were no major vascular complications with the X-Site device, whereas the frequency of major vascular complications with MC use in diagnostic procedures and PCI were 1.1% and 3.4%, respectively [11]. This represents the only preliminary randomized trial of any device that showed a decrease in vascular complications when compared with MC.

Sealant closure devices

Sealant devices have the longest history of effective hemostasis. The concept is to enhance the body's natural method of achieving hemostasis by delivering a procoagulant, such as collagen or thrombin, extravascularly to the surface of the femoral artery. Collagen and thrombin attract and activate platelets and form a quick coagulum at the surface of the artery and in the tissue tract that results in a seal. Unlike the suture-mediated closure devices, the sealant devices do not allow for immediate reaccess at the same arterial puncture site because of potential disruption of the sealant itself or potential embolization of the sealant into the femoral artery.

Angio-Seal closure device

Because of its incredibly simple design and deployment, the Angio-Seal (St. Jude Medical, Minneapolis, Minneapolis) VCD has become the most popular VCD in the United States, and represents more than 60% of the VCD market share. It works by a combination of mechanical forces and placement of a collagen plug that stimulates thrombus formation and platelet aggregation. Mechanically, it uses a "sandwich technique" at the arteriotomy site with an anchor on the intravascular side and a collagen plug on the extravascular side.

All cases require a predevice femoral angiogram to rule out PVD and to confirm femoral artery sheath placement. The original Angio-Seal device was cumbersome. It consisted of four components within a single carrier in an 8F package: the anchor, the connecting suture, the collagen plug, and a postplacement spring. Deploying the device is simple. First the artery is located when blood rushes out of the sheath and signifies that the sheath distal end is in the femoral arterial lumen. The dilator is removed and the carrier device is introduced into the sheath; this sets the anchor and introduces a 15-mg collagen sponge. A tamper is pushed downward to compress the collagen against the outer femoral arterial wall, the postplacement spring is attached between the tamper, and a metal tag is fixed to the positioning suture while applying continuous pressure on the tamper. All components are bioabsorbable within 90 days.

Because there was difficulty placing the post-collagen spring and there were reports of malalignment of the anchor that led to cessation of blood flow, embolization of the anchor itself, and inadvertent entry of the collagen sponge into the artery, the earlier Angio-Seal devices never proved to be popular. A series of iterations occurred over the last 5 years, including the introduction of the Millenium Platform that incorporated a monofold sheath design. This allowed for the use of a 6F sheath in place of the original 8F design.

The next iteration was revolutionary. The STS (self-tightening suture) Platform eliminated the need for a postplacement spring, which makes deployment incredibly simple and ensures an almost 100% success rate. Furthermore, it produced a more secure anchor–collagen sandwich. A single operator can deploy the device in less than 1 minute when proficient. The newest generation, the STS Plus, uses a smoother transition from sheath tip to dilator and has repositioned the blood inlet holes so that locating the artery is ensured once initial blood flow is seen. There is no need to enter, exit, and reenter the artery as was necessary with the original STS Platform.

The current Angio-Seal system is simple and effective. Successful deployment is seen in almost 100% of cases. Time to hemostasis is in the range of 2 to 4 minutes. The FDA allows for patient ambulation 20 minutes after diagnostic procedures. The author's laboratory has discharged patients home safely 1 hour after Angio-Seal closure. Immediate reaccess 1 cm above the original puncture site has been approved. Early reports showed a minor complication rate of 5.9% and major complication rates of 0.4% to 1.3% in PCI patients [12]. The author's laboratory has deployed more than 3000 Angio-Seal devices in patients who required PCI with a major complication rate of less than 0.4% (mostly retroperitoneal bleeds). The 6F device can close up to 8F sheaths and an 8F device is able to close up to 10F sheaths (Fig. 2).

Vasoseal closure device

Vasoseal (Datascope Corp.) represents the original sealant device. Originally introduced in 1995, this device consists of an entirely extravascular bovine collagen plug that induces the formation of a hemostatic cap above the puncture site in the tissue tract. The collagen is biodegradable and induces platelet aggregation, which releases coagulation factors and stimulates fibrin production and thrombus formation. The collagen reabsorbs by way of macrophages and

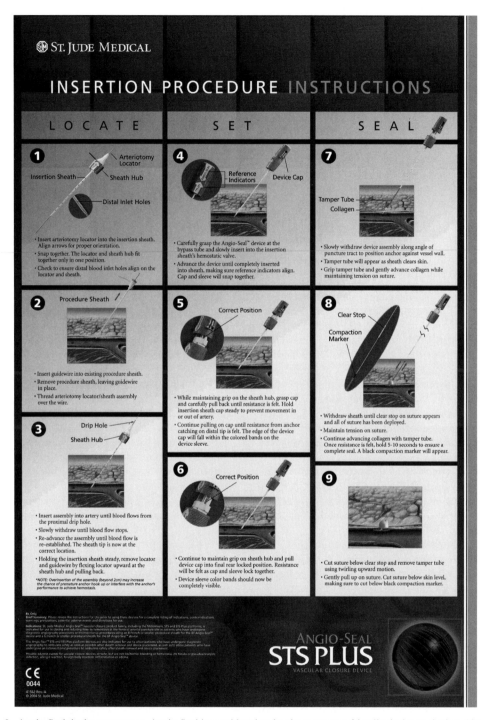

Fig. 2. Angio-Seal deployment steps. Angio-Seal is considered to be the most user-friendly device to deploy. (Courtesy of St. Jude Medical, Minneapolis, MN.)

granulocytes over a 6-week period. Because the device does not leave a foreign body inside the artery, it can be used in patients who have peripheral vascular disease. Additionally, no femoral angiogram is needed, which is a unique feature among VCDs.

The original Vasoseal VHD consisted of four parts: an 11F dilator, 11.5F sheaths of seven different lengths that were selected after a preprocedure needle depth technique was performed, and two 90-mg collagen cartridges. Placing this device required two people. First a guidewire was inserted into the femoral sheath and the sheath was removed while maintaining MC. A blunt-tipped 11F dilator was inserted over the wire to the site of the arterial puncture. The predetermined 11.5F sheath was advanced over the dilator down to the arterial surface. The dilator and wire were removed while the second operator held manual pressure from above. Finally, the collagen cartridge was deployed with a "push and pull" method through the sheath, and the sheath was removed. Light MC is then applied for a few minutes.

Recent iterations include the Vasoseal ES, which eliminated the need to premeasure arterial depth and the need for multiple 11.5F sheaths. It is approved for closure of 5F to 8F arterial sheaths. The Vasoseal Low Profile system was introduced more recently. This was a new, smaller device that was designed to be compatible with smaller sheaths (including 4F systems). The collagen plug was reduced by 40% and the delivery system was reduced by 3F sizes. Most recently, the Vasoseal Elite was launched with the promise of more rapid and effective hemostasis because of new collagen plug technology that allows for the immediate radial expansion of the plug that secures the collagen within the tissue tract within seconds of deployment in the tract. Vasoseal Elite reportedly no longer requires light MC after deployment and is effective in anticoagulated patients after PCI.

Clinical studies have demonstrated consistently decreased time to hemostasis compared with MC, usually within 5 to 8 minutes of deployment, in patients who undergo diagnostic procedures or PCI. The time to ambulation also is decreased significantly compared with MC; patients are able to ambulate safely at 1 hour after diagnostic procedures. Complications, such as infection, can occur from leaving a foreign body in the tissue tract. Minor local complications have been reported in approximately 8% of patients,

whereas major complications average approximately 5% in patients who undergo PCI [13]. Unfortunately, a large tissue tract is required to deploy the device, and if it fails to deploy the operator is left with a large tissue tract in an anticoagulated patient. This can lead to a large increase in vascular complications if the device fails to achieve hemostasis immediately. Because of the uncertainty in efficacy, especially when compared with Perclose or Angio-Seal, the Vasoseal device has not been able to capture a large market share, despite its unique feature of not leaving intra-arterial material at the end of the procedure.

Duett closure device

Duett (Vascular Solutions) is a newer sealant device that uses a combination of collagen and thrombin. It leaves no intra-arterial material and works solely by generation of a thrombus at the arterial puncture site. It has the advantage of leaving perhaps the least amount of inflammation after deployment but has the disadvantage of the possibility of a catastrophic complication—injecting thrombin/collagen mixture into the femoral artery or having the mixture leak into the femoral artery. It is easy to recognize this complication because it leads to an acutely ischemic leg almost immediately.

A femoral arteriogram should be obtained to rule out PVD and to ensure placement of the sheath in the common femoral artery. The Duett system uses a low-profile balloon-positioning catheter that goes over a core wire after the sheath is removed. When the device is inflated, the balloon becomes elliptical and provides temporary sealing of the arterial puncture site from inside. The balloon does allow for antegrade flow of blood in the artery during inflation so ischemia does not occur during balloon inflation. A mixture of 250 mg of bovine microfibrillar collagen and 10,000 units of bovine thrombin is made by the operator, and is injected slowly above the arterial puncture site through the side arm of the catheter. Almost immediate hemostasis is achieved and the patient usually feels a strong burning sensation as the procoagulant mixture is injected. The balloon is deflated and the catheter is removed from the patient. Because of the potency of the mixture, oozing is a rare complication after Duett closure. Immediate re-access is acceptable if the new puncture site is above the just closed arterial site.

Initial trials showed a success rate of 98% to 100%. Time to hemostasis and time to ambulation were decreased significantly compared with MC. Trials in patients who underwent diagnostic procedures or PCI showed a minor vascular complication rate of about 2% with a major complication rate of 1% [14]. Unfortunately, there is a 0.4% chance of inadvertent intra-arterial injection of the procoagulant mixture into the femoral artery that requires emergent therapy (Angiojet thrombectomy, intra-arterial infusion of thrombolytics, surgical thrombectomy). Because of the fear of this catastrophic complication, the Duett market share has been low.

A similar balloon occlusion system, called the Matrix, is to be released soon; it uses polyethylene glycol as the procoagulant. This has the advantage of being water soluble, and thus, dispersible, if injected into the arterial lumen. Trials are underway to investigate its clinical efficacy.

Staple-mediated closure devices

In the operating room, surgeons are now using staple technology at an increasing rate as a means for hemostasis over sutures. Staples can create an anatomic "purse-string suture" closure by using pledgets to gather vessel adventitia and media at the arteriotomy edges; this allows for tissue approximation and hemostasis. This technique is so effective that decannulation of large-bore cannulas from the ascending aorta is followed by a "purse-string suture" closure technique by way of large staples. This extraluminal closure does not impinge on intraluminal flow and does not leave any intra-arterial materials. Hence, one can use this device in patients who have PVD and in patients in whom the arterial puncture is below the femoral artery bifurcation.

The Angiolink vascular closure system (Medtronic, Santa Rosa, California) has received FDA approval as the first staple-mediated closure device. It consists of three components: a low-profile, 3-mm titanium staple; a one-piece "three-step" introducer assembly that contains an introducer, a dilator with a blood-marking lumen proximally, and two small stabilization filaments that stabilize the vessel wall during staple deployment; and a trigger-activated staple-deployment device.

To deploy the device, a guidewire is introduced into the arterial sheath before it is removed. The dilator and introducer are placed over the wire until blood is seen in the blood-marking lumen.

The wire is removed and the "three-step" introducer stabilizes the anterior vessel wall. The dilator is removed and the staple device is advanced through the introducer until the staple reaches the level of the anterior wall. As the trigger is activated, the staple is deployed into the media and adventitia of the femoral wall, the stabilization filaments are retracted, and the introducer is removed all at once (Fig. 3).

The Angiolink trial that led to FDA approval showed an in-hospital major complication rate of 0.4% versus 1.7% for MC. It is one of the few studies to show a decrease in complication rates compared with MC [15]. Of note, 80% of these patients received heparin and glycoprotein IIB/IIIA inhibition.

The Starclose (Abbott Vascular Devices) just received FDA approval and has been launched nationwide to much enthusiasm. It rivals the Angio-Seal device in simplicity and ease of use; it can be used in patients who have PVD or delivered in low sticks below the femoral artery bifurcation because of its extraluminal design. It delivers a nitinol clip between the media and adventitia, and thereby, leaves no material inside the arterial lumen. Oozing can be an issue because

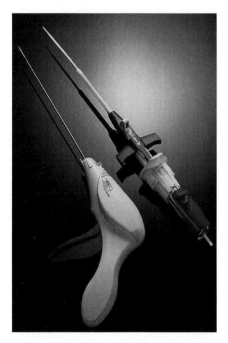

Fig. 3. Angiolink Staple Device. The first staple-mediated closure device. (Courtesy of Medtronic, Santa Rosa, CA.)

of the need to have a 7F tissue tract for the device to deliver the clip. There have been no reported cases of infection although real-world experience is not available. The Clip Closure in Percutaneous Procedures study randomized 208 patients who underwent diagnostic catheterization to Starclose or MC, and showed a mean time to hemostasis of 17 seconds and 15 minutes, respectively, and a mean time to ambulation of 4 hours and 6 hours, respectively [16]. If future studies show equivalent efficacy for hemostasis and low complication rates for the staple-and-clip technology, the use of suture-mediated and sealant closure devices may become obsolete (Fig. 4).

Do vascular closure devices lead to more complications?

Almost every trial has shown that VCDs decrease the time to hemostasis and the time to ambulation, and thereby, increase patient comfort and improve catheterization laboratory efficiency; however, because each device leaves behind foreign material (clip, sealant, suture), infection is always an increased concern. Because of the cost of VCDs (~$200–$250 for each device), overall safety and cost-effectiveness must be confirmed for most laboratories to invest in their usage.

The safety issue is controversial. Dangas and colleagues [17] reported that in the early experience with the first generations of VCDs, vascular complications were twice as common compared with MC, especially the frequency of surgical repair, hematoma formation, and the large hematocrit drop. This finding is probably due to the difficulty in placing these devices and the unfamiliarity of the devices to most operators at that

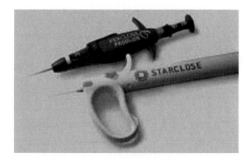

Fig. 4. The recently approved Starclose nitonol clip device. The new Starclose device may replace the popular Perclose suture-mediated closure device. (Courtesy of Abbott Vascular, Redwood City, CA.)

time. Each device has its own learning curve; if one becomes proficient in a certain device, vascular complications become less common.

Koreny and colleagues [18] published a large meta-analysis of more than 30 randomized trials (>4000 patients) that reported an increased risk for hematoma and pseudoaneurysm with the use of VCDs. This trial looked at a heterogenous patient population over a long period of time and probably was flawed by the use of earlier versions of the devices and the lack of operator comfort.

More recent data showed better results for VCDs when more recent devices were used. Meyerson and colleagues [19] reported no difference in the frequency of obtaining vascular surgical consults when VCDs were compared with MC in 4800 patients. Resnic and colleagues [20] studied more than 3000 patients in their institutional registry who underwent PCI; most patients were closed with Angio-Seal. There was a decrease in the rate of vascular complications in the device arm (3% versus 5.5%) and a 1-day decrease in hospital length of stay (2.8 versus 4.0 days). These indicate the cost effectiveness of these devices if they decrease hospital complications that lead to an increased length of stay. Applegate and colleagues [21] similarly showed an overall decrease in the rate of minor and major vascular complications (1.5% versus 2.5% with MC) when Perclose was used in 80% of nearly 4800 patients who underwent PCI. This again shows how the frequency of vascular complications is low when operators are familiar with a particular device.

The data from the Mt. Sinai School of Medicine, where more than 9000 patients have undergone PCI (55% Perclose and 45% Angio-Seal), show a significant decrease in pseudoaneurysms, arteriovenous fistulas, and large hematomas compared with MC [22]. This has led to a decrease in hospital length of stay. Each patient who receives a VCD is reprepped partially with new towels and new gloves. Diabetics and obese patients receive a dose of antibiotics. This has led to almost no cases of device infection.

Summary

VCDs have become a mainstay in high-volume cardiac catheterization laboratories because of their ability to decrease time to hemostasis and ambulation. It is obvious from patients who remember the days of only MC that they are satisfied with their more recent experiences with

VCDs. It cannot be overemphasized that only a laboratory that becomes dedicated in the use of VCDs and trains a small number of individuals to place a large number of certain VCDs can succeed in demonstrating a low rate of vascular complications that justifies their usage.

Although the efficacy and relative ease of deployment has pushed Angio-Seal and Perclose to the top of the field today, the newer staple-and-clip technologies may become the wave of the future for their simplicity and ability to close almost any patient.

References

[1] Meyerson SL, Feldman T, Desai TR. Angiographic access site complications in the era of arterial closure devices. Vasc Endovasc Surg 2002;14:652–6.

[2] Carey D, Martin JR, Moore CA, et al. Complications of femoral artery closure devices. Catheter Cardiovasc Interv 2001;52:3–7.

[3] Strategic growth opportunities in cardiovascular interventional treatment drives cardiology sector, American Health Consultants. BBI Newsletter 2001; 5:1–6.

[4] Seldinger SI. Catheter replacement of the needle in percutaneous arteriography. Acta Radiol 1953;39: 366–76.

[5] Najjar SF, Healey N, Healey CM, et al. Evaluation of poly-N-acetyl glucosamine as a hemostatic agent in patients undergoing cardiac catheterization: a double-blind, randomized study. J Trauma 2004; 57(1 Suppl):S38–41.

[6] Nader RG, Garcia JC, Drushal K, et al. Clinical evaluation of SyvekPatch in patients undergoing interventional, EPS, and diagnostic cardiac catheterization procedures. J Invasive Cardiol 2002;14: 305–7.

[7] Alter BM. Noninvasive Hemostasis Pad. Endovascular Today 2005;April:60.

[8] Fisher TH, Connolly R, Thatte HS, et al. Comparison of structural and hemostatic properties of the poly-N-acetyl glucosamine Syvek Patch with products containing chitosan. Microsc Res Tech 2004; 63:168–74.

[9] Vetter J, Ribeiro E, Hinohara T, et al. Suture mediated percutaneous closure of femoral artery access sites in fully anticoagulated patients following coronary interventions. Circulation 1994;90:I-621.

[10] Carere RG, Webb JG, Ahmed T, et al. Initial experience using Prostar: a new device for percutaneous suture-mediated closure of arterial puncture sites. Catheter Cardiovasc Diagn 1996;37:367–72.

[11] Sanborn TA, Ogilby JD, Ritter JM, et al. Reduced vascular complications after percutaneous coronary interventions with a nonmechanical suture device: results from the randomized RACE study. Catheter Cardiovasc Interv 2004;61:327–32.

[12] Cremonesi A, Castriota F, Tarantino F, et al. Femoral arterial hemostasis using the Angio-Seal system after coronary and vascular percutaneous angioplasty and stenting. J Invas Cardiol 1998;10: 464–9.

[13] Sanborn TA, Gibbs HH, Brinker JA, et al. A multicenter randomized trial comparing a percutaneous collagen hemostasis device with conventional manual compression after diagnostic angiography and angioplasty. J Am Coll Cardiol 1993;22:1273–9.

[14] Mooney MR, Ellis SG, Gershony G, et al. Immediate sealing of arterial puncture sites after cardiac catheterization and coronary interventions: initial US feasibility trial using the Duett vascular closure device. Catheter Cardiovasc Interv 2000;50: 96–102.

[15] Caputo RP, Ebner A, Grant WG, et al. Percutaneous femoral arteriotomy repair: initial experience with a novel staple closure device. J Invas Cardiol 2002;14:652–6.

[16] Hermiller J, Simonton C, Hinohara T, et al. Clinical experience with a circumferential clip-based vascular closure device in diagnostic catheterization. J Invasive Cardiol 2005;17:504–10.

[17] Dangas G, Mehran R, Kokolis S, et al. Vascular complications after percutaneous coronary interventions following hemostasis with manual compression versus arteriotomy closure devices. J Am Coll Cardiol 2001;38:638–41.

[18] Koreny M, Riedmuller E, Nikfardjam M, et al. Arterial puncture closing devices compared with standard manual compression after cardiac catheterization: systematic review and meta-analysis. JAMA 2004;291:350–7.

[19] Meyerson SL, Feldman T, Desai TR. Angiographic access site complications in the era of arterial closure devices. Vasc Endovasc Surg 2002;36(2): 137–44.

[20] Resnic FS, Blake GJ, Ohno-Machado L, et al. Vascular closure devices and the risk of vascular complications after percutaneous coronary intervention in patients receiving glycoprotein IIb/IIIa inhibitors. Am J Cardiol 2001;88:493–6.

[21] Applegate RJ, Grabarczyk MA, Little WC, et al. Vascular closure devices in patients treated with anticoagulation and IIb/IIIa receptor inhibitors during percutaneous revascularization. J Am Coll Cardiol 2002;40:78–83.

[22] Kim MC, Kini AS, Lee PC. Arterial closure devices decrease vascular complications after percutaneous coronary interventions. J Am Coll Cardiol 2004;43: A53.

**ELSEVIER
SAUNDERS**

Cardiol Clin 24 (2006) 287–297

**CARDIOLOGY
CLINICS**

Quality Management and Volume-Related Outcomes in the Cardiac Catheterization Laboratory

Richard L. Snider, MD, Warren K. Laskey, MD*

*Department of Medicine, Division of Cardiology, University of New Mexico School of Medicine,
MSC 10-5550, 1 University of New Mexico, Albuquerque, NM 87131, USA*

Quality in the cardiac catheterization laboratory (CCL) environment can be viewed as the end result of a dynamic interaction among numerous factors encompassing clinical, procedural, technical, cognitive, and process-related elements. Although procedural "outcomes" are the most conspicuous and increasingly relied-on measure of quality, it is essential to understand that such outcomes are a complex and composite mix of the previously noted general elements. Given the dependence of quality (and outcomes) on these elements, the assessment of quality may be viewed in quantitative terms as the output of a model whose independent and, it is hoped, scalable covariates account for most of the variance in the dependent variable (ie, quality). The assessment of quality, its control, and the effort to improve quality when the latter is perceived as a continuous process can be viewed in much the same way as their counterparts in industry [1,2]. It is unfortunate that the variability in human disease and human performance—key covariates in any model—continue to elude precise definition and quantification.

The identification of quality as the principal focus in the CCL environment [3,4] and the standards and processes necessary to achieve and improve quality have been described in detail [5,6]. The purposes of the present discussion are (1) to review the factors identified as necessary elements of quality in the CCL; (2) to review current approaches to the assessment of quality (of outcomes) in the CCL; (3) to discuss the applications, implications, and limitations of current means of assessing quality of outcomes in the CCL; and (4) to outline areas where there is need for additional information to more precisely quantify this elusive variable.

An understanding of the use of outcomes as a potentially quantifiable measure of quality posits a consensus regarding terminology and a comprehensive assessment of the factors contributing to such outcomes. Regarding the former, it is unfortunate that there is substantial variation in definitions of outcomes that reflects the heterogeneity of the evidence base (ie, observational cohort studies, randomized controlled clinical trials, post hoc retrospective analyses, and so forth). Outcome data obtained from safety-oriented clinical trials are more likely to include or emphasize traditional "hard" end points (eg, death, stroke, myocardial infarction [MI]), whereas outcome data obtained from efficacy-oriented clinical trials are more likely to include "softer" end points (eg, repeat revascularization, repeat hospitalization). Although there is unanimity regarding the hierarchic categorization of (adverse) clinical outcomes—death followed by MI followed by emergent coronary bypass surgery, and so forth—there is less agreement regarding the proper place of more recently recognized adverse sequelae of catheter-based procedures such as postprocedural cardiac biomarker detection and contrast-associated nephropathy. There is also substantial variation in agreement regarding the time window of ascertainment of outcomes (eg, in-hospital, postdischarge, 30 days). Such variability in the ascertainment of the dependent variable (outcome) presents its own obvious set of difficulties regarding an association (or

---

* Corresponding author.

E-mail address: wlaskey@salud.unm.edu
(W.K. Laskey).

lack thereof) with important exposure variables (see later discussion). Thus, in studies or approaches to the assessment of quality in the CCL, a clear and consistent definition of the outcome is essential. The overwhelming majority of outcome studies from the CCL environment focus on adverse outcomes that have a low frequency, which often presents insurmountable statistical issues [7]. Curiously, the reporting of beneficial outcomes is seldom found in the quality and outcome literature for the CCL.

Among the numerous factors contributing to CCL outcomes, operator-specific elements (technical competency, clinical judgment, cognitive base) and patient-specific elements (clinical presentation, lesion characteristics) have received the most scrutiny [8]. Additional important (although less well studied) contributions to outcomes arise from the "facility" and the continuous quality improvement process (Table 1). The number and the diversity of these factors underscore the critical importance of estimating risk-adjusted outcomes [9], notwithstanding the potential imprecision of this estimate owing to lack of transportability of models over time or geography [10–12]. Most studies have focused on in-hospital mortality or a composite major adverse clinical event rate as the outcome variable of interest; however, low event (mortality) rates remain a significant limitation to meaningful interpretation and extrapolation of these models to other settings [10,11]. In addition, the use of standardized mortality rates is subject to similar limitations owing to instability of the denominator (which is derived from such models).

It is unfortunate that there is a paucity of literature analyzing the comprehensive relationship between the elements outlined in Table 1 and the composite end point of in-hospital adverse

Table 1
Factors contributing to clinical outcomes in the cardiac catheterization laboratory

Operator-specific	Patient-specific	System/process - specific
Competency/technical proficiency	Demographic features	Institutional volume
Experience base	Clinical features	Clinical QA/CQI process
Cognitive base	Lesion features	Technical QA/CQI process

Abbreviations: CQI, continuous quality improvement; QA, quality assessment.

outcomes (death/MI/coronary bypass surgery/stroke). As these latter measures of outcome continue to improve [13], the earlier-noted limitations of mortality-centered models will also extend to these latter models. For this reason, several investigators have proposed using adverse outcome rates at 30 days [10,14,15], although no models incorporating the variables from Table 1 have been examined in this setting. Further complicating this issue is the absence of scalable covariates that capture the full dimensions of the "process" or "system" pieces.

Recently, the addition of procedural volume (institutional and operator-specific) has been added to the list of covariates in statistical models of CCL procedural outcomes [16,17]. Although attractive by virtue of its immediacy and simplicity, rigorous study of the accuracy, validity, and incremental value of this parameter to the classic risk- adjusted models of procedural outcome is lacking. Nevertheless, the currently accepted association between procedural volume (operator level and institutional level) and outcome is increasingly used as an index of (if not a surrogate for) quality and therefore deserves careful analysis.

The volume–outcome relationship

Historically, the relationship between procedural volume and clinical outcome has been attributed to the idea that "practice makes perfect." A wide variety of health care–related treatment strategies and procedures have been evaluated, including those related to cancer and HIV, congenital and acquired cardiac disease, and peripheral vascular disease. The data extracted from these studies have become the subject of much interest for health insurance purchasers, public consumers of health care, hospital administrators, and state regulators.

The surgical experience

The relationship between surgical procedural volume and clinical outcome has been extensively evaluated. As early as 1979, Luft and colleagues [18] examined clinical outcomes of 12 different surgical procedures varying in complexity. Mortality rates were reduced when open heart and coronary artery bypass graft (CABG) surgery, vascular surgery, or transurethral resection of the prostate were performed in centers that had an experience of greater than 200 procedures per year compared with lower-volume institutions.

More recently, large population–based studies have demonstrated a reduced mortality rate in higher-volume centers compared with lower-volume centers [19–21]. The magnitude of difference and the threshold at which these differences are seen are variable among different procedures. For example, surgical mortality was studied in the Medicare population using Medicare Provider Analysis and Review files from the Center for Medicare and Medicaid Services from 1994 through 1999 [21]. Analysis performed on 14 different surgical procedures showed improved observed and adjusted mortality rates for higher-volume compared with lower-volume centers. The largest adjusted differences in mortality rates were seen in patients undergoing pancreatic resection (16.3% versus 3.8%), esophagectomy (20.3% versus 8.4%), and pneumonectomy (16.1% versus 10.7%) when very low volume and very high volume centers were compared. The smallest difference between low- and high-volume centers was seen in the group undergoing carotid endarterectomy (1.7% versus 1.5%).

The percutaneous transluminal coronary angioplasty experience

The first studies evaluating the volume–outcome relationship within the realm of percutaneous coronary intervention (PCI) included patients undergoing percutaneous transluminal coronary angioplasty (PTCA) (Table 2). In 1989, Ritchie and colleagues [22] analyzed outcomes following PTCA in over 24,000 patients in nonfederal hospitals in California. Unadjusted in-hospital mortality was similar in admitted patients who had acute MI (AMI) or who did not have AMI among low-, intermediate-, and high-volume institutions. The unadjusted same-stay CABG rate and the composite rate of same-stay CABG or death (for the AMI and non-AMI groups), however, were significantly lower in the high-volume institutions.

Jollis and colleagues [23] analyzed a large dataset of Medicare beneficiaries from 1987 to 1990 and found that in-hospital and 30-day mortality rates and same-stay CABG rates declined when highest to lowest deciles of hospital PTCA volume were compared. These differences remained significant after adjustment for age, sex, race, and year of procedure. Individual operator and hospital volumes were analyzed when the Medicare population was studied again in 1992 [24]. There was no in-hospital or 30-day mortality difference as annual physician volume increased, but the rates

of same-stay CABG were higher in the low-volume group. Hospital volume remained a statistically significant risk factor for mortality and CABG, although the differences among volume groups were smaller compared with what was seen in the earlier report [23].

Examination of the Society for Cardiac Angiography and Interventions registry allowed Kimmel and colleagues [25] to collect detailed clinical patient information and thereby further adjust for differences among the volume strata. Despite the low overall rates for death and emergency CABG, a volume-dependent variation in outcomes was seen. A statistically significant decrease in the composite end point of death, emergency CABG, and postprocedural MI in laboratories performing more than 400 procedures per year was present compared with those performing fewer than 400. When multivariable logistic regression models were used to adjust for clinical characteristics (eg, chronic renal insufficiency, emergency PTCA, left main angioplasty, and shock, which were all more common in lower-volume centers; and congestive heart failure, recent MI, and complex lesion morphology, which were all more common in higher-volume centers), a statistically significant difference in emergency CABG, MI, and composite of major complications remained.

Hannan and colleagues [26] analyzed the relationships between hospital volume or individual operator volume and clinical outcomes by extracting data from the Coronary Angioplasty Reporting System (CARS). This system contains clinical information that is more detailed than what is found in administrative datasets. The study, which included over 60,000 patients undergoing PTCA in New York State from 1991 to 1994, found statistically significant higher risk-adjusted rates of mortality and same-stay CABG in the lowest hospital volume and lowest individual volume groups compared with the state as a whole. Further analysis indicated that high-volume operators working in high-volume centers tended to have improved outcomes compared with low-volume operators working in high-volume centers.

Experience in the current (stent) era

With advances in technology and pharmacology, there has been a decline in rates of postprocedural MI, CABG surgery, and in-hospital mortality [27–30]. The effect of these new therapies on the volume–outcome relationship has

Table 2
Percutaneous transluminal coronary angioplasty volume–outcome studies

Study [ref.]	Year/population studied	Data source	Unit of analysis (no. in group)	Definition of volume (cases per year)	Outcome (overall event rate)	Effect size: lowest-minus highest-volume group[a]
Ritchie et al, 1993 [22]	1989 multicenter	Administrative	Hospital (110)	Low (<200) High (>400)	In-hospital mortality (1.4%) Same-stay CABG (5%)	0.9% in AMI 0.0% in non-AMI 3.7% in AMI 1.9% in non-AMI
Jollis et al, 1994 [23]	1987–1990 multicenter	Administrative	Hospital (1194)	Deciles Low (<47) High (>371)	In-hospital mortality (2.9%) 30-day mortality (3.2%) In-hospital CABG (3.8%)	1.4% 1.5% 2.5%
Jollis et al, 1997 [24]	1992 multicenter	Administrative	Hospital (984) and individual (6115)	Physician Low (<25) High (>50) Hospital Low (<100) High (>200)	In-hospital mortality (2.5%) 30-day mortality (2.9%) Same-stay CABG (3.3%)	Physician: 0.1% Hospital: 0.6% Physician: 0.1% Hospital: 1.0% Physician: 1.2% Hospital: 0.9%
Kimmel et al, 1995 [25]	1992–1993 multicenter	Clinical	Hospital (48)	Low (<200) High (≥600)	In-hospital mortality (0.25%) Emergency CABG (1.3%)	0.2% 0.7%
Hannan et al, 1997 [26]	1991–1994 multicenter	Clinical	Hospital (31) and individual (not available)	Quintiles Physician Low (<75) High (≥250) Hospital Low (<400) High (≥1000)	In-hospital mortality (0.90%) Same-stay CABG (3.43%)	Physician: 0.06%[b] Hospital: 0.17%[b] Physician: 0.87%[b] Hospital: 0.95%[b]

Abbreviation: AMI, acute myocardial infarction.
[a] Rates presented are the unadjusted difference between the lowest and highest volume for the outcome shown unless otherwise specified.
[b] Risk adjusted difference.

been addressed in single and multicenter studies (Table 3).

Kastrati and colleagues [31] evaluated outcomes in 3409 consecutive patients who underwent coronary stent implantation performed by 10 different operators in a single center from 1992 to 1997. Using a composite end point of cardiac death, MI, or CABG at 30 days post procedure, the investigators found that compared with the overall event rate, operators performing greater than 483 procedures annually had better outcomes, whereas operators performing less than 90 procedures annually had worse outcomes. Using a classification and regression tree analysis, the investigators also found that minimum procedural volume appeared to be a determinant of outcome, even for patients who had less complex lesion types.

Data from larger multicenter samples such as the Medicare population and information from the National In-Patient Sample (NIS) have also been published. McGrath and colleagues [32] examined individual and hospital volume and the relation to outcome for over 167,000 Medicare patients who underwent PCI in 1997. The difference in crude rates of CABG between high- and low-volume hospitals became nonsignificant when adjustment was made for clinical risk factors; however, a difference in 30-day mortality favoring high-volume centers persisted. When physician volume was examined, differences in crude 30-day mortality became statistically insignificant when outcomes were adjusted for risk; however, a difference in risk-adjusted rates of CABG occurred in favor of high- versus low-volume strata. Investigators from an NIS-based study [33] compared high- versus low-volume centers and demonstrated a statistically significant decrease in in-hospital mortality of patients who did and did not have AMI in 1997. Analysis of the same database over the interval from 1998 to 2000 showed a similar trend in mortality benefit in high-volume centers [34]. No difference in risk-adjusted in-hospital mortality was found, however, when intermediate-volume centers (performing 200–399 annual PCIs) were compared with those performing more than 400 annual PCIs.

In a recent study from a high-volume (>4000 interventional procedures per year) institution from 1999 to 2001, no association between operator volume and adverse outcomes (crude and risk-adjusted in-hospital death and the composite of death, CABG surgery, MI, or stroke) could be identified [35]. These latter findings are similar to an earlier publication by the Northern New England Cardiovascular Disease Study Group [36] that showed that there was no statistical difference in risk-adjusted in-hospital mortality, same-stay CABG, MI, or clinical success among terciles of operator volume. Centers included in this study performed greater than 600 procedures per year.

The acute myocardial infarction experience

Risk-adjustment models have been used to correct for differences in patient characteristics that may affect crude rates of outcome and their association with volume. Patients presenting with AMI are a high-risk group, with overall higher rates of in-hospital death compared with patients who present with stable coronary syndromes. Although many studies of the volume–outcome relation have included patients who have AMI in their analyses, few have looked at this patient population exclusively (Table 4).

Using information from the Cooperative Cardiovascular Project, Thiemann and colleagues [37] noted that in 98,898 Medicare patients treated with primary angioplasty, thrombolysis, or conservative medical management for AMI, crude and risk-adjusted 30-day mortality rates were lower in the highest-volume quartile compared with the lowest-volume quartile. In addition, analysis of medical therapy received by the different groups showed a higher use of aspirin, β-blockers, and other appropriate pharmacologic therapies in the higher-volume groups, which accounted for about one third of the difference in outcome.

Vakili and colleagues [38] analyzed the CARS database in 1995 and found that when hospital volume was divided into terciles, there was no correlation between volume and in-hospital mortality for crude or risk-adjusted outcome in patients undergoing primary angioplasty for AMI. A lower mortality rate, however, was noted in the highest tercile of individual procedural volume compared with the lowest. When the same patient population was reanalyzed, but the categorization of individual procedural volumes was changed to correlate with current American College of Cardiology/American Heart Association recommendations (<75 cases per year considered low individual volume; <400 cases per year considered low hospital volume), individual volume did not have an effect on in-hospital mortality, and high-volume hospitals had a statistical advantage over low-volume

Table 3
Stent-era volume–outcome studies

Study [ref.]	Stents used in PCI	Year/ population studied	Data source	Unit of analysis (no. in group)	Definition of volume (cases per year)	Outcome (overall event rate)	Effect size: lowest-minus highest-volume group[a]
Kastrati et al, 1998 [31]	100%	1992–1997 single-center	Clinical	Individual (10)	Quintiles Low (<90) High (>242)	30-day combined cardiac death, MI, CABG (2.99%)	2.5%
Malenka et al, 1999 [36]	Nearly 50% by 1996	1994–1996 multicenter	Clinical	Individual (47)	Terciles Low (22–84) High (≥138)	In-hospital mortality in Low risk (NA) High risk (NA) Same-stay CABG (NA)	−0.26% −1.55% 0.47%
Watanabe et al, 2002 [33]	59%	Only 1997 data presented here multicenter	Administrative	Individual (NA)	Low (≤200) High (> 400)	In-hospital mortality in AMI (3.5%) Non-AMI (0.8%) Same-stay CABG in AMI (2.9%) Non-AMI (1.8%)	1.7% 0.2% −0.4% 0.4%
McGrath et al, 2000 [32]	48.4%–61.1%	1997 multicenter	Administrative	Hospital (1003) and individual (6534)	Individual[b] Low (<30) High (> 60) Hospital[b] Low (<80) High (> 160)	30-day mortality (3.30%) Same-stay CABG (1.87%)	Individual: −0.14% Hospital: 1.14%[c] Individual: 0.70% Hospital: 0.0%[c]
Epstein et al, 2004 [34]	81.7%	1998–2000 multicenter	Administrative	Hospital (457)	Low (<200) Intermediate (200–399) High (400–999) Very high (≥1000)	In-hospital mortality (1.58%)	1.2% (low-minus very high volume group) 0.19% (intermediate minus high-volume group)
Harjai et al, 2004 [35]	71%	1999–2001 single-center	Clinical	Individual (28)	Terciles Low (<93) High (>140)	In-hospital mortality (0.99%) Composite death, MI, CABG, CVA (2.59%)	−0.22% 0.11%

Abbreviations: CVA, cerebrovascular accident; NA, not available.
[a] Rates presented are the unadjusted difference between the lowest and highest volume for the outcome shown unless otherwise specified.
[b] Low and high volumes correspond to individual volumes of <75 and > 150 and hospital volumes of <200 and >400 if estimated Medicare volume is 40% of total volume.
[c] Risk adjusted difference.

Table 4
Primary angioplasty volume–outcome studies

Study [ref.]	Year/population studied	Data source	Unit of analysis (no. in group)	Definition of volume (cases per year)	Outcome	Effect size: lowest-minus highest-volume group[a]
Vakili et al, 2001 [38]	1995 multicenter	Clinical	Hospital (32) and individual (151)	Terciles Individual Low (1–10) High (≥11) Hospital Low (1–56) High (≥57)	In-hospital mortality	Individual: 3.3%[b] Hospital: 1.8%[b]
Vakili et al, 2003 [39]	1995 multicenter	Clinical	Hospital (32) and Individual (151)	Individual[c] Low (<75) High (≥75) Hospital[c] Low (<400) High (≥400)	In-hospital mortality	Individual: 1.3%[a] Hospital: 3.8%[b]
Magid et al, 2000 [40]	June 1, 1994–July 31, 1999 multicenter	Clinical	Hospital (446)	Low (<16) High (≥49)	In-hospital mortality (1° angioplasty) Thrombolysis	2.8% 0.5%
Canto et al, 2000 [41]	June 1994–March 1998 multicenter	Clinical	Hospital (450)	Quartiles Low (5–11) High (>33)	In-hospital mortality (1° angioplasty) Thrombolysis	2.0% −0.1%
Tsuchihashi et al, 2004 [42]	1997 multicenter	Clinical	Hospital (129)	Terciles Low (1–16) High (56–370)	In-hospital mortality Same-stay CABG	1.0%[b] 0.9%[b]

[a] Rates presented are the unadjusted difference between the lowest and highest volume for the outcome shown unless otherwise specified.
[b] Multivariate risk adjustment did not change statistical outcome.
[c] Categories are based on total annual PTCA volume shown in parentheses for individual and hospital; number of primary angioplasties not available.

hospitals [39]. Statistical significance remained when mortality rates were risk adjusted.

Using the National Registry of Myocardial Infarction (NRMI) database from June 1994 through July 1999, Magid and colleagues [40] compared in-hospital mortality in over 62,000 patients presenting with AMI treated with primary angioplasty or thrombolytic therapy as a function of hospital primary angioplasty volume. Mortality rates were significantly lower in the intermediate- and high-volume centers for patients who underwent primary angioplasty compared with those who underwent thrombolysis. Low-volume centers, however, demonstrated no difference in mortality when these two treatment modalities were compared. Although no direct statistical comparison of outcome was made among the low-, intermediate-, and high-volume hospitals in the primary angioplasty group alone, there was a trend toward decreasing in-hospital mortality with increasing volume. Other investigators in the NRMI registry [41] collected data from June 1994 to March 1998 and found an association between in-hospital mortality and hospital volume in patients undergoing primary PCI for AMI. Crude and risk-adjusted mortality rates were lower in the highest-volume quartile compared with the lowest-volume quartile. These investigators could not demonstrate an association between hospital volume and mortality when thrombolytic therapy was used as the reperfusion strategy. In 1997, investigators of the Japanese Coronary Intervention Study [42] evaluated 2491 patients who underwent PCI for AMI and found no difference in crude or risk-adjusted in-hospital mortality rate or same-stay CABG rate among terciles of hospital volume.

Longitudinal studies

A decline in overall risk-adjusted mortality and same-stay CABG rates from 1990 to 1997 was noted in a report from the Northern New England Cardiovascular Disease Study Group [30]. Trends in improving clinical success rates of PCI, MI, and same-stay CABG were seen across the 8-year period in unadjusted and risk-adjusted rates despite a concomitant increase in the prevalence of risk factors (eg, age, diabetes, renal failure, previous CABG, and left main disease). Although this study was not designed to evaluate physician or hospital volume, the investigators contended that the improved outcomes were related, in part, to an increase in physician and hospital volume, with the most significant contribution being from technologic advances.

As rates of adverse outcomes continue to decline along with improvements in operator skill and technology, the magnitude of the difference in outcomes between high-and low-volume groups is likely to diminish. An analysis of procedural outcomes in California addresses the volume–outcome relationship among low-, intermediate-, and high-volume facilities over time [43]. Files from the Office of Statewide Health Planning and Development in California were reviewed, and data were extracted from charts of 353,488 patients who were admitted after undergoing coronary intervention between 1984 and 1996. A trend in decreasing mortality and CABG rates was seen as procedure volume increased; however, the magnitude of difference among the different volume groups decreased over time (Fig. 1). This finding was true for crude and risk-adjusted rates. Fig. 2 shows that with the addition of more recent data from Epstein and colleagues [34], the difference in mortality when comparing intermediate-volume (200–399 cases per year) to high-volume (≥400 cases per year) centers continues to decrease over time. Centers performing fewer than 200 cases per year, however, continue to demonstrate higher mortality rates [34].

Summary

In this article, the authors have attempted to summarize the factors necessary for the comprehensive assessment of quality and outcomes in the CCL environment. The focus has been on the

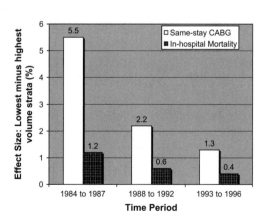

Fig. 1. Diminishing differences in outcome between low-volume (<200 cases per year) and high-volume (≥400 cases per year) centers in California over time. (*Data from* Ho V. Evolution of the volume-outcome relation for hospitals performing coronary angioplasty. Circulation 2000;101:1806–11.)

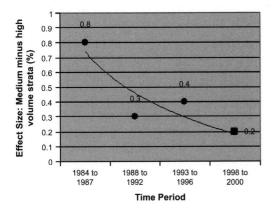

Fig. 2. Time-dependent changes in the difference in mortality between intermediate-volume (200–399 cases per year) and high-volume (≥400 cases per year) categories. (*Data from* Ho V. Evolution of the volume-outcome relation for hospitals performing coronary angioplasty. Circulation 2000;101:1806–11 and Epstein AJ, Rathor SS, Volpp KG, et al. Hospital percutaneous coronary intervention volume and patient mortality, 1998 to 2000. Does the evidence support current procedure volume minimums? J Am Coll Cardiol 2004;43: 1755–62.)

association between outcome measures and procedural volume and on the methodologies used in such studies; however, the authors have also introduced a note of caution into unhesitating acceptance of the quality-outcomes-volume syllogism. Although there is, overall, a statistically significant association between procedural outcomes and volume, the magnitude of this association is highly dependent on (1) the type and frequency of the outcome; (2) the clinical setting; (3) the nature of the measuring instrument (administrative versus clinical database); (4) the unit of analysis (individual operator versus institution); (5) the effects of temporal changes in clinical practice and outcomes; (6) the cut points used to define volume; (7) the robustness and transportability of risk-adjustment models (for prediction of outcomes); and (8) system and process considerations.

Although the use of clinical outcomes as an indicator of quality is certainly reasonable, outcome assessment alone does not capture the universe of the elements of quality or aid us in understanding the processes of quality control and quality improvement. The latter should be highly visible and "real." A closely related question is, If we could impact one of the more important aspects of the process of care in the

CCL, would we favorably alter outcomes? One study suggests so [44], and the impact on outcomes demonstrated, for the first time, that such efforts have meaningful sequelae. Many more studies of a similar nature under widely varying clinical, demographic, and temporal conditions will be required before we are ready to accept procedural outcomes as the sole measure of quality. Similar concerns arise regarding the use of procedural volume as a surrogate of quality. As discussed herein, there is sufficient variability in the measures currently used to assess this relationship such that considerable circumspection is advised for the unwary. The importance of the definition of volume is underscored by sequential studies from the CARS registry [38,39] of the volume–outcome relationship in patients undergoing PCI for AMI. Using the same patient population but varying the cut points for low and high volume, these studies demonstrated discordant conclusions regarding a volume–outcome relationship.

Finally, given the interstudy variation in the extent of an association between volume and outcome and the decreasing absolute magnitude of difference in outcomes across quantiles, the inability to embrace fully a quality-outcome-volume syllogism must be acknowledged. A greater appreciation of the merits and limitations of the methodology used to analyze the association between volume and outcomes is needed. All such associations derived from observational studies must be scrutinized for the effects of confounding and bias because the latter may certainly influence (positively or negatively) the measure of that association. Furthermore, given the diminishing absolute differences in mortality across strata of volumes and the ever-increasing size of datasets, the question of statistical versus clinical relevance assumes greater importance. Certainly, from a population-based perspective, small percentage differences multiplied across a large sample size will result in a significant number of patients overall. The extension of these population-based data to the individual patient becomes problematic. From an individual perspective, such small percentage differences may be difficult to translate into clinical relevance.

References

[1] Grant E, Leavenworth R. Statistical quality control. 7th edition. New York: McGraw Hill; 1966.

[2] Available at: http://www.ge.com/sixsigma/SixSigma/ pdf. Accessed July 1, 2005.

[3] Sones FM Jr. The Society for Cardiac Angiography. Cathet Cardiovasc Diag 1978;4:233–4.

[4] Hildner FJ. Quality is the only issue. Cathet Cardiovasc Diag 1990;3:216–7.

[5] Bashore TM, Bates ER, Berger PB, et al. Cardiac catheterization laboratory standards: a report of the American College of Cardiology Task Force on Clinical Expert Consensus Documents (ACC/ SCAI committee to develop an expert consensus document on catheterization laboratory standards). J Am Coll Cardiol 2001;37:2170–214.

[6] Society for Cardiac Angiography and Interventions. Monograph on quality management in the cardiac catheterization laboratory. Bethesda (MD): SCAI; 1999.

[7] Ellis SG, Omoigui N, Bittl JA, et al. Analysis and comparison of operator-specific outcomes in interventional cardiology: from a multi-center database of 4860 quality-controlled procedures. Circulation 1996;93:431–9.

[8] Hirshfeld JW Jr, Ellis SG, Faxon DP, et al. Recommendations for the assessment and maintenance of proficiency in coronary interventional procedures: statement of the American College of Cardiology. J Am Coll Cardiol 1998;31:722–43.

[9] Block PC, Peterson EC, Krone R, et al. Identification of variables needed to risk adjust outcomes of coronary interventions: evidence-based guidelines for efficient data collection. J Am Coll Cardiol 1998;32:275–82.

[10] Hannan EL, Wu C. Assessing quality and outcomes for percutaneous coronary intervention: Choosing statistical models, outcomes, time periods and patient populations. Am Heart J 2003;145: 571–4.

[11] Kizer JR, Berlin JA, Laskey WK, et al. Limitations of current risk-adjustment models in the era of coronary stenting. Am Heart J 2003;145:683–92.

[12] Holmes DR, Selzer F, Johnston JM, et al. Modeling and risk prediction in the current era of interventional cardiology. Circulation 2003;107:1871–6.

[13] Williams DO, Holubkov R, Yeh W, et al. Percutaneous coronary intervention in the current era compared with 1985–86: the National Heart, Lung and Blood Institute Registries. Circulation 2000;102: 2945–51.

[14] Lindsay J, Pinnow EE, Pichard AD. Benchmarking operator performance in percutaneous coronary intervention: a novel approach using 30-day events. Cathet Cardiovasc Interv 2001;52:139–45.

[15] Laskey WK, Selzer F, Jacobs AK, et al. Importance of the post-discharge interval in assessing major adverse clinical event rates following percutaneous coronary intervention. Am J Cardiol 2005;95:1135–9.

[16] Phillips KA, Luft HS, Ritchie JL. The association of hospital volumes of percutaneous transluminal coronary angioplasty with adverse outcomes, length of stay and charges in California. Med Care 1995; 33:502–14.

[17] Hannan EL, Racz M, Ryan TJ, et al. Coronary angioplasty volume-outcome relationships for hospitals and cardiologists. JAMA 1997;277:892–8.

[18] Luft HS, Bunker JP, Enthoven AC. Should operations be regionalized? The empirical relation between surgical volume and mortality. N Engl J Med 1979;301:1364–9.

[19] Hannan EL, O'Donnell JF, Kilburn H Jr, et al. Investigation of the relationship between volume and mortality for surgical procedures performed in New York State hospitals. JAMA 1989;262:503–10.

[20] Finlayson EV, Goodney PP, Birkmeyer JD. Hospital volume and operative mortality in cancer surgery: a National Study. Arch Surg 2003;138:882–90.

[21] Birkmeyer JD, Siewers AE, Finlayson E, et al. Hospital volume and surgical mortality in the United States. N Engl J Med 2002;346:1128–37.

[22] Ritchie JL, Phillips KA, Luft HS. Coronary angioplasty: statewide experience in California. Circulation 1993;88:2735–43.

[23] Jollis JG, Peterson ED, DeLong ER, et al. The relation between the volume of coronary angioplasty procedures at hospitals treating Medicare beneficiaries and short-term mortality. N Engl J Med 1994; 331:1625–9.

[24] Jollis JG, Peterson ED, Nelson CL, et al. Relationship between physician and hospital coronary angioplasty volume and outcome in elderly patients. Circulation 1997;95:2485–91.

[25] Kimmel SE, Berlin JA, Laskey WK. The relationship between coronary angioplasty procedure volume and major complications. JAMA 1995;274: 1137–42.

[26] Hannan EL, Racz M, Ryan TJ, et al. Coronary angioplasty volume-outcome relationships for hospitals and cardiologist. JAMA 1997;277(11):892–8.

[27] Kimmel SE, Localio AR, Krone RJ, et al. The effects of contemporary use of coronary stents on in-hospital mortality. Registry Committee of the Society for Cardiac Angiography and Interventions. J Am Coll Cardiol 2001;37(2):499–504.

[28] Maynard C, Wright SM, Every NR, et al. Comparison of outcomes of coronary stenting versus conventional coronary angioplasty in the department of veterans affairs medical centers. Am J Cardiol 2001;87:1240–5.

[29] Use of a monoclonal antibody directed against the platelet glycoprotein IIb/IIIa receptor n high-risk coronary angioplasty. The EPIC Investigation. N Engl J Med 1994;330:956–61.

[30] McGrath PD, Malenka DJ, Wennberg DE, et al. Changing outcomes in percutaneous coronary interventions. A study of 34,752 procedures in northern New England, 1990 to 1997. J Am Coll Cardiol 1999;34:674–80.

[31] Kastrati A, Neuman FJ, Shomig A. Operator volume and outcome of patients undergoing

coronary stent placement. J Am Coll Cardiol 1998; 32:970–6.

[32] McGrath PD, Wennberg DE, Dickens JD, et al. Relation between operator and hospital volume and outcomes following percutaneous coronary interventions in the era of the coronary stent. JAMA 2000;284:3139–44.

[33] Watanabe CT, Maynard C, Ritchie JL. Short-term outcomes after percutaneous coronary intervention: effects of stenting and institutional volume shifts. Am Heart J 2002;144:309–14.

[34] Epstein AJ, Rathor SS, Volpp KG, et al. Hospital percutaneous coronary intervention volume and patient mortality, 1998 to 2000. Does the evidence support current procedure volume minimums? J Am Coll Cardiol 2004;43:1755–62.

[35] Harjai KJ, Berman AD, Grines CL, et al. Impact of interventionalist volume, experience, and board certification on coronary angioplasty outcomes in the era of stenting. Am J Cardiol 2004;94:421–6.

[36] Malenka DJ, McGrath PD, Wennberg DE, et al. The relationship between operator volume and outcomes after percutaneous coronary interventions in high volume hospitals in 1994–1996. J Am Coll Cardiol 1999;34:1471–80.

[37] Thiemann DR, Coresh J, Oetgen WJ, et al. The association between hospital volume and survival after acute myocardial infarction in elderly patients. N Engl J Med 1999;340:1640–8.

[38] Vakili BA, Kaplan R, Brown DL. Volume-outcome relation for physicians and hospitals performing angioplasty for acute myocardial infarction in New York State. Circulation 2001;104:2171–6.

[39] Vakili BA, Brown DL. Relation of total annual coronary angioplasty volume of physicians and hospitals on outcomes of primary angioplasty for acute myocardial infarction (data from the 1995 Coronary Angioplasty Reporting System of the New York State Department of Health). Am J Cardiol 2003; 91(6):726–8.

[40] Magid DJ, Calonge BN, Rumsfeld JS, et al. Relation between hospital primary angioplasty volume and mortality for patients with acute MI treated with primary angioplasty vs thrombolytic therapy. JAMA 2000;284:3131–8.

[41] Canto JG, Every NR, Magid DJ, et al. The volume of primary angioplasty procedures and survival after acute myocardial infarction. N Engl J Med 2000; 342:1573–80.

[42] Tsuchihashi M, Tsutsui H, Tada H, et al. Volume-outcome relation for hospitals performing angioplasty for acute myocardial infarction: results from the Nationwide Japanese Registry. Circ J 2004;68: 887–91.

[43] Ho V. Evolution of the volume-outcome relation for hospitals performing coronary angioplasty. Circulation 2000;101:1806–11.

[44] Moscucci M, Share D, Kline-Rogers E, et al. The Blue Cross Blue Shield of Michigan Cardiovascular Consortium (BMC2) collaborative quality improvement initiative in percutaneous coronary interventions. J Interv Cardiol 2002;15:381–6.

ELSEVIER
SAUNDERS

Cardiol Clin 24 (2006) 299–304

CARDIOLOGY
CLINICS

Index

Note: Page numbers of article titles are in **boldface** type.

Changing Your Address?

Make sure your subscription changes too! When you notify us of your new address, you can help make our job easier by including an exact copy of your Clinics label number with your old address (see illustration below.) This number identifies you to our computer system and will speed the processing of your address change. Please be sure this label number accompanies your old address and your corrected address—you can send an old Clinics label with your number on it or just copy it exactly and send it to the address listed below.

We appreciate your help in our attempt to give you continuous coverage. Thank you.

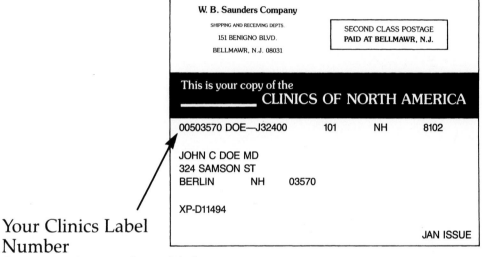

Your Clinics Label Number

Copy it exactly or send your label
along with your address to:
Elsevier Periodicals Customer Service
6277 Sea Harbor Drive
Orlando, FL 32887-4800
Call Toll Free 1-800-654-2452

Please allow four to six weeks for delivery of new subscriptions and for processing address changes.